Aging and Family Therapy: Practitioner Perspectives on Golden Pond

THE *JOURNAL OF PSYCHOTHERAPY & THE FAMILY* SERIES:

Aging and Family Therapy: Practitioner Perspectives on Golden Pond

George A. Hughston
Victor A. Christopherson
Marilyn J. Bonjean
Editors

The Haworth Press
New York • London

Aging and Family Therapy: Practitioners Perspectives on Golden Pond has also been published as *Journal of Psychotherapy & the Family*, Volume 5, Numbers 1/2 1988.

The Haworth Press, Inc. 10 Alice Street, Binghamton, NY 13904-1580
EUROSPAN/Haworth, 3 Henrietta Street, London WC2E 8LU England

Library of Congress Cataloging in Publication Data

Aging and family therapy : practitioner perspectives on golden pond / George A. Hughston,
   Victor A. Christopherson, Marilyn J. Bonjean, editors.
      p. cm.
      "Has also been published as Journal of psychotherapy & the family, volume 5, numbers 1/2,
1988" — T.p. verson.
      Includes bibliographies.
      ISBN 0-86656-778-X
      1. Aged — mental health. 2. Family psychotherapy. I. Hughston, George A. II. Christopher-
son, Victor A., 1923 –   . III. Bonjean, Marilyn J.
      [DNLM: 1. Aged — psychology, 2. Family Therapy. 3. Psychotherapy — in old age. W1
JO859C v: 5 no. 1/2 / WT 150 A2663]
RC451.4.A5A36   1989
155.67--dc19
DNLM/DLC
for Library of Congress
                                                                    88-39357
                                                                    CIP

Aging and Family Therapy: Practitioner Perspectives on Golden Pond

CONTENTS

ABOUT THE EDITORS

George A. Hughston, PhD, is Associate Professor and former Chair of the Department of Family Resources and Human Development, Arizona State University, Tempe. He has over 20 years of experience teaching, consulting, and counseling older people and their families. Dr. Hughston has made over 100 radio and television presentations, predominantly on adult development and aging. He is a co-author of *Counseling the Elderly: A Systems Approach* and a co-editor of *Independent Aging: Reading in Social Gerontology*. He earned a doctorate degree from Pennsylvania State University in human development and family studies with a major emphasis in gerontology. Dr. Hughston is an active member of the American Association of Professional Counselors, the Gerontological Society, and the National Council on Family Relations.

Victor A. Christopherson, EdD, is Director of the School of Family and Consumer Resources and Professor of Human Development, University of Arizona, Tucson. Dr. Christopherson, whose general areas of research include gerontology, rural and medical sociology, and socialization, is currently conducting research on personality continuity through the life span. He is the author of four books, a number of chapters in textbooks, and approximately 50 articles in professional journals. He has previously taught at the universities of California, Hawaii, and Connecticut.

Marilyn J. Bonjean, EdD, a clinical member and approved supervisor of the American Association for Marriage and Family Therapy, is in private practice at ICF Consultants, Inc., Milwaukee, Wisconsin, where she provides psychotherapy, consultation, and training regarding issues of chronic illness and clinical gerontology. She is a clinical faculty member of the University of Wisconsin-Milwaukee, School of Social Welfare and the University of Wisconsin Medical School, Department of Psychiatry, Sinai-Samaritan Clinical Campus. Dr. Bonjean has administered programs in long-term care institutions for the past 10 years and has served as a speaker and consultant for community programs. Dr. Bonjean's publications, which include *Something for the Family*, *Making Visits Count*, and *In Support of Caregivers*, provide guidance for those establishing educational supportive groups for caregivers of frail elderly.

EDITORIAL NOTE

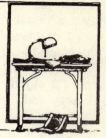

   This special journal issue, focusing on aging and family therapy, marks the final volume, Volume 5, of my tenure as Editor of the *Journal of Psychotherapy & the Family* and its co-published monograph editions. It is with great pleasure that the *Journal* and its monograph series welcomes this fine double issue. It has taken me nearly my entire tenure to locate such a fine editorial team to produce this collection. The *Journal* monograph series is dedicated to improving the arts and sciences of psychotherapy practice by focusing on the family and its role in the prevention, development, and maintenance of psychopathology. The aim of the *Journal* series is to provide the most well-written, accurate, authoritative, and relevant information on critical issues in the practice of psychotherapy with families. This *Journal* issue/monograph edition, consistent with the *Journal*'s aim, intends to promote new insight into the complex issues associated with providing family therapy services to this important and growing population.

   When I began to develop the founding concepts of this *Journal* and its monograph editions in 1983 I believed that the special topic of marriage and family therapy for elderly people was critically important. I never imagined it would be so difficult to finally bring such a collection to fruition. At that time, and now, there exists no book available to assist psychotherapists working with the elderly on marriage and family clinical issues. For the first time, this collection provides a comprehensive overview of these issues, edited by a nationally-known and experienced group of family gerontology therapists. The purpose of the collection is to offer the practitioner up-to-date information, insight, and reference sources that will enable the practitioner to provide more effective intervention with the elderly and their families. The authors promote a systemic strategy and illustrate its utility throughout.

This fine editorial team is headed by George A. Hughston. Dr. Hughston is Associate Professor of Family Studies, Arizona State University. Dr. Hughston has teaching and counseling experience at the Cedar Medical Center, Brigham Young University, the Pennsylvania State University, and Arizona State University. His journal publications are found in *Perceptual and Motor Skills, The International Journal of Aging and Human Development, Journal of Long-term Care and Health Services Administration, Journal of Psychology, Journal of Genetic Psychology, The Journal of Educational Psychology, Journal of Sex and Marital Therapy, Psychological Reports, Family Coordinator,* and *Development Psychology*. Dr. Hughston has long been a featured speaker at many national meetings, and maintains a high level of activity in local, state, and national organizations. His current community involvement includes work with the Arizona Parkinson's Institute, the Arizona Consortium for the Homeless, and the Arizona Department of Corrections. Among his many publications is the classic *Counseling the Elderly: A Systems Approach* (Harper & Row, 1981) co-authored with Dr. James Keller. Victor A. Christopherson is Professor of Family Studies, Univerisity of Arizona. The other co-editor, Dr. Marilyn J. Bonjean, is a clinical member and approved supervisor of the American Association for Marriage and Family Therapy, and is in private practice at Individual, Couple, and Family Consultants, Inc., Milwaukee. She teaches gerontology and family therapy at the University of Wisconsin-Milwaukee and has provided clinical gerontology services in long term care settings for over ten years. She serves as a grantswoman for supportive programs to elderly persons and their families, and as a speaker and consultant for community programs. Dr. Bonjean's publications in the area of family therapy and support to children of the aging have been widely used in support groups and educational programs. These include *Something for the Family*, *Making Visits Count*, and *In Support of Caregivers* which provide guidance for those establishing educational support- ive grousp for caregivers of frail elderly.

It is not surprising then, that this excellent editorial team was so successful in attracting papers and such an impressive list of con- tributors. Together, this collection suggests that systemic family therapists, equipped with knowledge about aged clients and sys- tems, are ideally suited to treat older adults and their families. The editors assert that this is so because these professionals ". . . are accustomed to thinking about problems in behaviorally descriptive terms, and they understand that solutions often require management of the interactions of complex variables."

Many psychotherapists believe that they are sufficiently prepared to work with the elderly and their family and that the same methods can be utilized with younger adults as well. I hope that these col- leagues will read this collection and discover, as I did many years ago, that this is just not true. For some of us, however, our anxiety about working with this special population is as much our prejudice and ageism, as it is ignorance. The practical side of this issue is, of course, that living means aging, as the death rate is decreasing and the average age of our population is increasing. Practicing psycho- therapists will be seeing more and more elderly clients. Thus, read- ing this collection of fine papers will become more of a necessity with time, albeit our more mature clients obviously deserve our full attention and sensitivity right now. Please let either one of the co- editors know what you think about this collection.

Happy reading and aging!

Charles R. Figley, PhD
Editor, *Journal of Psychotherapy & the Family*

Aging and Family Therapy:
An Introduction

George A. Hughston
Victor A. Christopherson
Marilyn J. Bonjean

A relatively new emphasis in family psychotherapy parallels that of geriatric medicine in its concern for maximizing the health and well being of older people. While "the" elderly are a relatively heterogenous group, covering an age span of 40 years or more, there are sufficient commonalities among the aged and their families to require specialized knowledge and treatment procedures by family therapists. Concerns that might bring the services of family practitioners into play are initiated by what could be termed "the issues of aging," including retirement, bereavement, ageism, mental or emotional illness, economic or money management, role transitions, sexual functions, addition, and others.

With expanding percentages of the population joining the ranks of old people, psychotherapy with the aged and their families represents a challenging new area of emphasis. This new frontier requires a working knowledge of the myths and realities which accompany the aging process. A systematic approach to the family will assist in understanding the ties relevant to successful psychotherapy.

The systematic context in which most problem behavior among the elderly occurs, is the family. When a family member is distressed in some fashion, other family members are also affected. Sympathy, knowledge, and insight among family members can have ameliorative influence, while a lack of these qualities can exacerbate the difficulties and generate hostility and alienation. Tension cycles build within a family system and spin out of control when the rational perspectives are lost and actors become embroiled in maladaptive dynamics. All ages, including the very young, will interact with these problem issues as they revolve within the family system. Intervention by a person skilled in systemic therapeutic techniques and endowed with knowledge of essential intervening difficulties can make a significant contribution to the restoration of equilibrium.

Current trends and projections indicate that increasingly larger proportions of the population will be effected by the issues of aging. The demand for psychotherapy with the elderly and their families can be expected to increase accordingly. Hopefully, practitioners will anticipate this need and prepare themselves accordingly.

As a step toward meeting this anticipated need, the editors have solicited original articles from outstanding scholars which address some major issues from the practitioner's vantage point. We feel that many of the articles are destined to become classics, and we feel privileged to offer them as "firsts."

PURPOSE AND OBJECTIVES

Providing successful psychotherapy for older adults and their families requires that practitioners restructure approaches to overcome objections elderly people generally have toward therapy. The present cohort of older adults is not "psychologically minded." They have experienced a more primitive mental health system and harbor fears of being declared insane and institutionalized. Even talking about private feelings or family matters to a stranger is an unfamiliar experience for many and may be seen as an admission of incompetence. Discussing problems with someone else may be especially frightening if it also increases feelings of dependency.

Successful treatment of older adults will be systemic in nature, that is, it will consider the context of the older adult as an organized whole with parts or subsystems continuously interconnected in a mutually regulatory, patterned relationship. The exchange of information and energy among the biological, psychological, social and spiritual domains of the aged will be examined so that all relevant information may be used to formulate a systemic and comprehensive treatment plan. This integrated systemic view allows the therapist to organize observations so that elements of physical and mental status, medication usage, intergenerational relationships, living environment, involvement of community service providers, financial resources, legal issues, societal stereotypes and role expectations may all be part of problem formation and solution. The therapist will assess the interplay among various component parts of these systems and use this information to plan intervention which impacts multiple systems and brings other service providers into alignment with therapeutic goals and interventions. This complex management of interacting systems makes treatment of older adults especially challenging.

A brief, solution-focussed approach will help older adults experience positive results from therapy rather quickly and enhance their commitment to the therapy process. An approach which assesses and adapts to the client's language, world view, and values is essential. By behaviorally describing problems occurring in the present and setting goals which, when achieved, are clearly credited to the client's efforts, anxieties will be allayed and results will be affirming to the older adult. The client can be free to express intimate feelings if comfortable doing so, but the emphasis is placed on behavioral changes.

Inclusion of the family or emotionally-significant-others in the therapeutic plan is important to successful outcomes. A majority of older adults have relatives and are in regular contact with them. Functional family relationships can support therapeutic intervention and prevent inappropriate institutionalization. Many families are searching for guidance in the new experience of multi-generational relationships. Such relationships become especially difficult if mental or physical impairment of an elder is an issue. Treatment which attempts to create a fit among the individual and family histories, qualitative relationships and coping capacities, and the needs of impaired relatives will develop solutions which endure over time.

As the increasing number of older adults raises the demand for mental health services to those in late life, family therapists will be called upon to provide assistance. Systemic family therapists are ideally suited to treat older adults and their families because they are accustomed to thinking about problems in behaviorally descriptive terms, and they understand that solutions often require management of the interactions of complex variables.

In summary, the purpose of this collection is to provide the practitioner with information, insight, reference sources and other tools that contribute to more effective intervention with the elderly and their families. A systemic strategy is utilized to illustrate appropriate therapeutic techniques throughout.

ORGANIZATION AND CONTENT

This collection includes papers contributed by professionals from disciplines related to effective therapeutic intervention with the elderly person and his or her family. Like a puzzle, each paper contains pieces of timely information which help create a completed picture basic to effective family therapy. Although most practicing therapists will be familiar with segments of each chapter, much new information will illustrate the growing importance of specific knowledge concerning older people and their families. Intervention strategies should be enhanced by each contribution.

The first paper, by Daniel S. Nieto, Raymond T. Coward and Donald L. Horsley, "Principles of Therapeutic Intervention with Elders and Their Families," encourages realization of the elusive goal of collaboration and coordination between the family and providers of services to the elderly. The authors emphasize the necessity to maximize strengths inherent within formal and informal helping networks through practitioner utilization of six principles guiding interaction. Therapists should benefit from this fresh view of categories which characterize the interactions of elderly people, their families and those involved in the helping professions. Examples are used to illustrate the six principles of ongoing assessment; ownership of locus of decision-making; interventive parsimony; clarification of perceptions, expectations and roles; levels of participation; and the use of professional authority. This chapter provides a foundation for both a theoretical and a practical basis for family treatment across approaches.

The next paper, by James F. Keller and Mark C. Bromley, "Psychotherapy with the Elderly: A Systemic Model," acknowledges the contextual nature of common problems faced by elderly people and their families as well as the values of utilizing a systemic strategy for effective therapeutic intervention. This innovative chapter includes an overview of traditional models while highlighting goals the practitioner may utilize in assessment of progress in the process of psychotherapy. The authors develop five strategies and techniques for presenting options with the elderly. The strategies include: emotional connections review; techniques for the family group meeting; the probe for strength; the world of counterpointing realities; and structured reminiscence. These strategies are followed by a case study which illustrates the implementation and application of the strategies.

The third paper by George A. Hughston and Nancy J. Cooledge is devoted to benefits gained from reflection upon the past. Individuals, families and their therapists may gain substantial insight into current behavior by reviewing perceptions of past experiences. Reminiscence by the aged and their families is proposed as a positive tool for systemic family intervention. For the experienced counselor, a substantial list of benefits may be gained from exploration of past family history. This chapter proposes that long-past family experiences may serve to enhance current activities which help erase the negative and enhance the positive. The work concludes with a list of suggestions for successful utilization of reminiscence.

The fourth paper reports "A Life Systems Approach to Understanding Parent-Child Relationships in Aging Families." The work, by Roberta Greene, emphasizes the necessity for involvement of the entire family in problem resolution, and the importance of the therapist's role as a mobilizer of the family system. The therapist is viewed as necessary in order to create positive interdependence as the adult child assumes additional responsibilities of providing care for elderly family members. Additional stress and strain will become evident throughout the family, affecting the young as well as the old. Emphasis throughout this paper is placed upon the effective use of intergenerational family therapy which involves mobilization of the family in order to resolve the problems of the aged. This paper also provides insight regarding clinical treatment methods from a systems perspective. Examples which clarify the treatment plan are provided in order to illustrate Greene's phases of applied family therapy. As one reviews this paper, it becomes increasingly evident that it is impossible for mental health professionals to ignore the later stages of life and the critical role the family therapist plays in dealing with parent-child relationships in aging families. For Greene, a family treatment orientation is vital to resolution of problems of the elderly and one of the major mental health challenges of the next decade.

The next paper, by Vicki L. Schmall and Clara C. Pratt, supplements previous papers by confronting the realities of dependency and the impact that declining abilities have upon families. In spite of well-meaning intent, families are victims of demographic and social trends which limit their abilities to be of service to their elderly members. Even the most warm, sensitive family members will lack resources to provide needed long-term support. Family members will experience stress, dilemmas and difficult decisions in providing care for the aged. Schmall and Pratt discuss four strategies that can enhance a family's effectiveness to make decisions and their ability to provide caregiving. The first strategy, educational programs, is viewed from a problem-solving, conflict-resolution point of departure rather than a traditional didactic presentation format. The second, family conferences, is offered as a solution which may assist early caregiving and create problem resolution strategies which may prevent onset of additional anticipated problems. The third, providing support which helps normalize the experience of caregivers through socially acceptable outlets may be viewed as therapeutic. Levels of burden may be shared and bonds of intimacy and support may be formed. The fourth strategy offered by this paper is respite service, i.e., temporary relief from caregiving responsibilities. Both the caregiver and the ill person may benefit from this outside-the-family socialization according to Schmall and Pratt.

The sixth paper, "Reversible Mental Illness: The Role of the Family in Therapeutic Context," by Gregory L. Schmidt, is devoted to the role families play in maximizing potential for reversal of mental illness. Caregiving strategies providing support, education and psychotherapy for family caregivers are viewed as critical factors which may prevent institutionalization as well as facilitate recovery from a range of psychiatric illness. The paper includes an overview of common psychiatric problems affecting the elderly, presents information regarding prevalence and etiology of these illnesses, and discusses approaches to treatment. Schmidt outlines former causes for the avoidance of psychiatric intervention with the elderly as he supports the necessity for renewed focus upon the family's role in recognition and understanding of a relative's psychiatric problems. Support from the family system is viewed as crucial to a psychotherapist's assistance with effective and successful intervention.

The seventh paper, "Caring for the Depressed Elderly and Their Families," was contributed by Richard McQuellon and Burton Reifler. This work is directed toward the area of the depressed elderly and their families through examination of models of depression from a variety of professional disciplines. Due to the past use of pluralistic approaches, the authors recommend multidisciplinary team strategies involving systemic diagnostic information. This paper effectively references depression inventories and somatic as well as non-somatic treatment approaches which have been found effective with this group. McQuellon and Reifler utilize case studies to illustrate a number of issues raised in the assessment and treatment of the depressed elderly. Throughout this paper, the systems approach is viewed as effective in overcoming definitional and diagnostic obstacles to the accurate assessment of depression. Current refinements in diagnostic criteria are listed for systemic therapists so they may maximize combined Family Centered approaches in releasing the healing properties in family ties.

The paper by Nancy Osgood, "A Systems Approach to Suicide Prevention," complements the previous paper. A major contribution is made as Osgood explores various factors which have been proven to contribute to suicide rates among the elderly. This insight is especially beneficial in viewing actual versus perceived risk among elderly clientele. Awareness is furthered by review of the cultural, social, and psychological explanation for higher suicide rates among this age group, a review which serves as a cornerstone for understanding preventive strategies. Viewed from a systemic perspective, the family is seen as a basic factor in health and illness, with direct ties between the individual state of mental health and the degree of health within the family. Family relationships may be viewed as a major source of stress, severe enough in some cases to result in suicide. Clues and warning signs of late-life suicide are presented as an in-depth discussion of the important role the family may play in prevention. The Osgood paper contributes to practitioner effectiveness through a detailed discussion of the practitioner role in working with the "at risk" individual and his/her family.

The ninth paper, "Roles of the Psychotherapist in Family Financial Counseling: A Systems Approach to Prolongation of Independence" by Richard Morse, presents an in-depth view of family financial counseling. Understanding both individual and family problems may include the often overlooked area of financial profiles. The financial profile provides the psychotherapist with the awareness and insight necessary to adequately evaluate current status and future provisions. Morse identifies a client's income, expenses, net worth, social support, rights, and claims to other persons and institutions as being of vital importance to mental health and well being. The family psychotherapist should be sensitive to and respect the limitations of the many individuals and families who have inadequate monetary support. Such individuals cannot utilize resources available to those more fortunate. If ever the statement, "Money may not buy happiness, but it may buy opportunity" is true, it is true with the aged. The Morse paper closes with a series of questions especially important to those older persons whose "count down" years become increasingly more finite.

The tenth paper, "Sexual Dysfunction in the Elderly: Causes and Effects" by James E. Garrison, views sexual expression among the elderly as a normal part of the aging process. With the exception of organic-related problems, sexual problems of the aged are viewed by Garrison to be quite similar to those of the young. This paper contributes to a more in-depth understanding of medication and health issues as related to the functional role sexuality plays in systemic therapy. In addition, insight is gained from a detailed discussion of therapeutic issues and options such as history taking, information sharing, and relationship problems. Many practitioners will benefit from Garrison's inclusion of resources for problem diagnosis and treatment.

The eleventh paper, "Legal Ramifications of Elderly Cohabitation: Necessity for Recognition of Its Implications by Family Psychotherapists" by Doryce Sanders Hughston and George A. Hughston, reviews the realities of cohabitation from a legal perspective. One's awareness of the impact law has upon the functions of effective individual and family relations cannot be over emphasized. Although detailed understanding of the law requires legal counsel, very basic questions are outlined in this paper. These basics serve to point out potential problem areas to the practitioner and may prevent future legal problems created by lack of awareness regarding cohabitation among the aged. For better or perhaps worse, the law is an integral part of the family system and invades systemic intervention. With increasing numbers of elderly people residing together out of wedlock, the family psychotherapist may assist clients by utilization of some of the directives provided within this paper.

Alcohol abuse is the next complex problem elaborated upon by Eloise Rathbone-McCuan and Jacquelyn Hedlund in paper twelve titled, "Older Families and Issues of Alcohol Misuse: A Neglected Problem in Psychotherapy." The paper extends insight through its distribution of recent information necessary for every practitioner touched by the issues related to alcohol misuse in later life. Three case studies are used to discuss risks to both long-term alcoholics who have grown old with their drinking problem and the risks confronting those who have only recently become a part of the alcohol addition spiral. The Rathbone-McCuan and Hedlund case studies well illustrate the crises nature of the differing consequences alcoholism creates within the family system. Major points include impact on separate family members and, also, on generations, requiring skilled family therapy with an alert systems focus. In conclusion, these authors present several principles of intervention and prevention which should be easily utilized by practitioners working with older persons and their families.

Paper number thirteen, "The Burden of Insight: A Basis for Constructive Response" by Victor A. Christopherson, is a reflective and thoughtful essay on a quality having great significance to human relationships. Christopherson joins Freud, Erickson and others who have recognized and considered the importance of insight to the quality of relationships. Insight is not a "given" that some have and some do not have, but a quality everyone can develop or increase. When one party in a relationship has more insight regarding relationship dynamics than the other has, the insightful individual carries a major burden for helping things go smoothly. Christ called it "going the second mile." Whereas there is much precedent for parent-child relationships in our society, the path for adult children who must assume a parent-like role for their parent is often unclear. The paper discusses the burden of insight from the vantage point of an adult child in a caregiving role. Two principal sources of conflict between the adult child and the elderly recipient, i.e., generational differences and senescence are illustrative of these problems. Issues of independence versus dependence, mortality versus morality, integration versus isolation, optimism versus pessimism, and resolution versus dissolution are discussed (Lewis and Lewis, 1986). The role of the adult child is considered within each type of conflict in order to optimize therapeutic outcome. It is critical for the adult child to understand both the normal decrements of senescence and their implications. In addition, it is important to understand those conditions which go beyond the normal such as chronic brain syndrome. The ability to distinguish between reversible and nonreversible conditions is necessary for effective systemic intervention.

Paper number fourteen by Marilyn J. Bonjean, "Solution Focused Psychotherapy with Families Caring for an Alzheimer's Patient," points to the reality of Alzheimer's disease as the fourth leading cause of death in the elderly and the potential impact this disease has upon the family system. An operating knowledge of this progressive and global impairment of the brain is of relevance to every practitioner working with the aged as it impacts the patient's family, communication patterns, roles, relationships, and family structure. Vast changes are required to accommodate care of this modified member of the family. Solution focused systemic strategic theory is proposed by Bonjean as a valuable foundation for intervention with families of Alzheimer's patients. A major contribution of this chapter includes the guidance of caregivers in creative planning appropriate and flexible enough to allow the needs of all family members to be met. A clear and precise understanding of the effects awaiting the Alzheimer's disease patient should clarify the unknown and greatly assist in family planning.

Neil G. McCluskey, co-editor of the recent book, *Retirement: Prospects, Planning, and Policy*, writes regarding the effects of

"Retirement and the Contemporary Family." McCluskey points out that an additional 27 years have been added to the life expectancy of children born in 1985 compared to those born in 1900. This increase has affected retirement patterns and families with elderly members. The paper discusses new ways to deal with these changes. A common perception of the elderly is that they are an increasingly costly consumer segment; a more accurate accounting should reflect their contributions as well. Many older people, for example, function as potential providers of services to the "old old" elderly. Sometimes these services, especially for the "young old" female, force critical decisions between retirement from the workplace in order to assume a more extensive caregiving role versus continuing to work in a capacity consistent with her abilities. McCluskey considers the term "retirement" to be inappropriate, preferring "transfer point" to more accurately reflect the change from roles from which one eventually withdraws to new roles assumed after the event. The McCluskey paper concludes with a rich description of community resources which the family caregiver may utilize. These resources are present in almost all communities and are described by the author as being important to adequately functioning family systems.

The concluding paper, number sixteen, "Bereavement and the Elderly: The Role of the Psychotherapist," is a comprehensive description of those parts of life including dying and bereavement. Death is a universal experience, yet one that confronts the practitioner with unusual stresses as he or she helps the dying as well as subsequently assisting those who have been bereaved as they deal with their losses and their grief. Williams uses Kubler-Ross's work as a launching point but identifies her five stages as symbolic of the dying experience rather than a lock-step process. The mechanisms of defense, the emotional stress, the needs and drives of the dying are just as unique and varied in the dying as in the non-dying. The paper utilizes a framework of analysis that is comprised of Endings, the Neutral Zone and New Beginnings with the healing journey through these processes taking from 18 months to as long as 4 years, and reviews four basic tasks to be completed by the bereaved. Williams provides techniques for the therapist to utilize in helping the bereaved, the dying individual, and the family to adjust to the loss.

Principles of Therapeutic Intervention with Elders and Their Families

Daniel S. Nieto
Raymond T. Coward
Donald L. Horsley

SUMMARY. Despite appeals for greater collaboration and coordination in the care of elders between family members and formal service providers, the realization of this goal has proven elusive. One element that appears to be critical to successful collaborative efforts is the ability of direct service providers to mediate between formal and informal networks and to mobilize the strengths inherent in each. In this context, six principles are offered to guide helping professionals in their interactions with elders and their families. Illustrations of the application of these practice principles in interventions with later life families are presented. The principles discussed are ongoing assessment; ownership or locus of decision-making; interventive parsimony; clarification of perceptions, expectations, and roles; levels of participation; and the use of professional authority. This set of principles is a starting point which, it is hoped, will stimulate further discussion and debate relative to those processes which characterize the interactions of practitioners with elders and their families.

INTRODUCTION

Despite the persistence of popular myths about families abandoning elders and abdicating their responsibilities for caregiving, research over the past decade has demonstrated repeatedly the promi-

Daniel S. Nieto, PhD, ACSW, is Assistant Professor of Social Work at The University of Vermont, Burlington, VT 05405-0160. Raymond T. Coward, MSW, PhD, is Professor and Director of the Social Work Program and Research Professor in the Center for Rural Studies at The University of Vermont. Donald L. Horsley, MSW, is a doctoral candidate in Administration and Planning at The University of Vermont.

nent and decisive involvement of family members in the care of elders (Brubaker, 1985; Cicirelli, 1981; Litwak, 1985; Sauer and Coward, 1985; Stephens and Christianson, 1986). Families provide care to elders in a variety of forms and under a number of different circumstances. There is evidence that family members are paramount in providing assistance, when needed, with both the most basic tasks of daily living such as eating, dressing, bathing or toileting (Stoller and Earl, 1983) as well as with a broader set of supportive activities such as managing money, shopping, housework or preparing meals (Coward, 1987; Van Nostrand, 1984). Moreover, family members are conspicuous among both those caregivers who live in the same household as dependent elders (Soldo and Myllyluoma, 1983) as well as those who provide support and assistance to elders who continue to live independently (Stephens and Christianson, 1986).

This is not to suggest that there is no limit to the care that can be, and is being, provided by families or that elders and their families should not, and do not, make use of the formal aid that is provided by social service agencies. Indeed, research has indicated that as age increases, as marital partners die and as health limitations intensify, it becomes more likely that elderly persons will be receiving simultaneously the help of both family members and formal care providers. Coward (1987) reported that 17.2% of a random sample of noninstitutionalized elders were utilizing simultaneously the services of both formal and informal helpers. For many of the most disabled and frail elderly and their families, it is not a question of "either/or" but, rather, a matter of identifying and defining the appropriate mixture and balance of family and formal caregiving.

The proposition that helping professionals need to be more aware of, and perhaps coordinate better, the relative contributions of family and formal caregivers is certainly not new. More than two decades ago Litwak (1965) introduced the concept of "shared functioning" and argued that the availability of both formal and informal support systems enhanced significantly the quality of life of older persons. More recently, however, concerns about the rapidly escalating cost of publicly financed services for the elderly, combined with absolute funding reductions in the overall public welfare sector, have intensified the attention that is being given to programs that are designed to coordinate, or to enhance, the collaboration between family and formal caregiving (Callahan, 1980; Stephens and Christianson, 1986).

While the concept of closer collaboration and coordination is an ideal that most formal and informal caregivers are eager to support, many have found it easier to articulate than to operationalize. Those elders and their families who have tried to "reach out" and join forces with the formal sector have often found it to be a confusing maze of programs, eligibility requirements, waiting lists, and provider-specific needs assessments (Horsley, 1985; Thornton and Dunston, 1986; Wood and Estes, 1985). Simultaneously, while the principle of collaboration with the family is an ideal that most formal service providers find consistent with their professional training, it can be a principle that is difficult, time consuming, and frustrating to incorporate into practice (Biegel, Shore and Gordon, 1984). There have been a number of service coordination models put forth and tested during the last fifteen years. Whether they were called case-management, care-management, or service-management, their common goal was to forge a collaboration between formal and informal caregivers that would lead to the more effective and efficient delivery of services to the elderly (Brown and Drake, 1980; Center for the Study of Social Policy, 1982; Horsley et al., 1980; Steinberg and Jurkiewicz, 1980). In each of these efforts, however, it has become apparent that, to be successful, direct service providers must have a set of practice skills which allows them to blend and mix the family and the formal service networks into a coherent whole and to capitalize on the strengths that lie within each system (Graham, 1984; Sager, 1982; Strong, 1981). Otherwise, the collaborative efforts, however structured, will fail.

In the sections below, we offer a set of principles that can be used by service providers to guide their efforts to create collaborative relationships between elders, families and formal service providers. This list is not meant to be an exhaustive, comprehensive enumeration of all the precepts necessary to guide gerontological practice or to provide guidelines for every conceivable situation that clients will present. Rather, in an effort to stimulate further discussion and debate, this list is a preliminary attempt to articular the overarching principles that should guide the interactions of practitioners with elders and their families. In addition, our goal is to begin to bridge what we see as a gap between the standard operating procedures of an established area of practice, family therapy, and the emerging practice context of later life families.

PRINCIPLES OF PROFESSIONAL/FAMILY INTERACTION

In the text that follows, we describe and discuss six principles to guide helping professionals in their interactions with later life families. There is little, if any, disagreement among professional practitioners involved in the treatment of families about the viability of these concepts as basic operating principles. While considerable variation exists with respect to the specific techniques and interventions that can be used with particular population groups, this set of principles provides both a theoretical and a practical basis for family treatment across approaches.

Ongoing Assessment

The first operating principle is that of joint (i.e., professional helper and client/client system) comprehensive, continuing assessment (Devore and Schlesinger, 1987; Hartman and Laird, 1983; Loewenberg, 1983). Rational planning requires that the practitioner becomes intimately familiar with both the client and the interactions of that client with the social and physical environments in which they exist. In reality, however, given the constraints of professional practice, not everything can be known at once. Assessment, therefore, must be conceived of as an incremental process that augments, on a continuing basis, what is known about the client. Assessment is, as a result, the step in the treatment process where such information as is available is studied, analyzed, and used as a basis for action, treatment, or intervention. Compton and Galaway (1984) emphasized the basic nature of this part of the helping process as follows:

> This process involves the ordering and organizing of the information, intuitions, and knowledge that client and worker bring so that the pieces come together into some pattern that makes sense, at least in the here and now, in explaining the problem and in relating this explanation to alternative solutions. (p. 397)

Assessment is, moreover, a part of the intervention process that pervades the course of client-professional interactions. Assessments must be on-going, continuous, and always subject to modification. Human beings, and their interactions with their environments, are not static; rather, they are always changing. Because they are dynamic, a static assessment makes little or no sense, except in that rare environment from which no further information can be elicited. However, because the eduction of some social services providers presents the helping process as if it were a series of discrete stages, there is a tendency among novice helping professionals to operate from an almost rigid ordering or sequencing of actions. As a consequence, the dynamic nature of human beings can be overlooked and assessment techniques can be developed that seem to be based on the assumption that interactions cease once initial contacts and an early assessment have been completed. Pincus and Minahan (1973) underlined this danger as follows:

> A pitfall in this process is the temptation for the worker to hold on to his initial assumptions and try to make the facts fit them, rather than the other way around. Knowing when and how to alter initial assumptions is essential to the exercise of professional judgement. It is helpful for the worker to keep in mind competing hypotheses and assumptions as new information becomes available, because the problem assessment is not a static assessment but changes as the planned changed [sic] process proceeds. Though it acts as an initial guide for the planned change process, it is a blueprint that is modified and detailed as the process proceeds. (p. 103)

Assessment is an essential early step in intervention. However, if the continuous, ongoing nature of assessment is overlooked, the potential effectiveness of ensuing interventions can be compromised. The necessity for ongoing assessment is particularly relevant when working with later life families. For example, we know that spouses, who are themselves elderly, are often the "first line of defense" for disabled and dependent persons over the age of 65 years (Hess and Soldo, 1985). Because their own abilities are subject to deterioration, and their own health needs may change dramatically, the capacity of such spouses to provide care is likely to change over time. Only with a system of ongoing assessment will practitioners be able to make appropriate modifications in care plans as these changes occur. Similarly, a significant number of adult children who are caring for elderly parents are themselves over 65 years of age (Brody, 1985). Such offspring are often coping with their own declining faculties or may be adjusting to changes in their own lifestyles such as retirement or widowhood. Whatever the individual circumstances, the capacity of elderly offspring to provide long term care to their parents may be altered with time. Only with a system of continuous assessment will practitioners be able to help elders, and families, make smooth transitions into new care plans as conditions change and as the "social convoys" of elders become recast (Depner and Ingersoll, 1980).

It should be stressed, further, that assessment should focus not only on the identified client but, in the ideal, on all of the significant members of the client's social support system. As Pincus and Minahan (1973) have characterized the process, "the worker should not view a problem as the property of a given person or persons, but as characteristic of their interactions" (p. 105). Care plans that involve clients, family members, friends, and others must, necessarily, be based on an ongoing, continuous assessment of the resources which reside in the various elements.

The levels of motivation, opportunity, and capacity of both the elder and the family support networks are the basis for intervention. Thus, interventions based on less than a thorough awareness of these elements are, conceptually, inadequate. The degree to which the client, for example, wants to be involved in his or her own treatment; the intellectual, emotional, physical, economic, and other resources which the client can bring to the treatment situation; and, the opportunities and resources available in the environment of the client must be known and evaluated relative to their potential utility in a care plan. Similarly, those aspects of the client system which are outside the identified client must be assessed, re-assessed, evaluated, and, if appropriate, utilized.

Clearly, not all elders are alike. Some will want to be actively involved in the creation of a care plan and, indeed, will be resentful and will act contrary to a plan developed without their full participation. In other cases, elders will have lost the mental capacity to participate meaningfully or will be experiencing such severe physical ailments that they are unable to function appropriately in such discussions. Whatever the individual circumstances, the goal must be, always, to maximize the participation of the elder in the development of a care plan. Such participation, incidentally, must be genuine and offered in earnest and should not be fabricated or feigned.

Ownership of the Decision-Making Process

Decision-making, relative both to planning and carrying out an intervention, must be viewed as "belonging" to the client system in much the same way that the problem constellation being addressed must be owned by the client system. The decision-making roles of the professional helper, therefore, are limited to those areas which the client and others in his or her environment are unwilling or unable to address. The role of professional helpers in assisting clients in making decisions is not diminished, however, as a result of the application of this principle. Rather, the skills and techniques required to provide such assistance *increase* the demands placed on the professional helper; and, as a consequence, the acquisition of these skills becomes increasingly important.

Elders and their families often come into contact with professional helpers at a time of personal crisis, e.g., an elderly woman, living alone, who needs help recuperating from a broken hip; a widower whose chronic illness means that more and more outside help will be needed if he is to remain in his own apartment; or, an adult child who reaches a point of complete exhaustion and feels unable to continue providing care to his or her elderly parent. In each of these events, the professional caregiver will need to take the utmost care in avoiding the tendency of some elders and family members to relinquish all decision-making to the expert (Brandt et al., 1982; Brown and Drake, 1980). The family may welcome the professional's "taking charge" and telling them what they should do. Certainly there will be instances where such a style of operation could be justified—but it should be the exception and *not* the rule. There is simply too much evidence and research that demonstrates the importance of elders' actively participating in decisions about their care (Biegel et al., 1984). The process of collaboration must include investing decision-making, to the degree possible, in clients and their families.

Parsimony

When alternative intervention options exist, in the ideal, the most parsimonious, and least disruptive, intervention should be considered to be the approach of choice (Loewenberg, 1983). Those activities which are least disruptive of the "normal" activities of the client are to be preferred to those which may appear to be potentially more efficient but which are more complex and tend to remove the client from familiar physical and psychological routines. The professional helper can be of assistance to clients and families in assessing the degree of disruption that will result from a given intervention and can aid the client system in maintaining a realistic frame of reference for exploring, developing, and choosing from among alternative courses of action.

For elders, and their families, adherence to this principle has often involved attempts to keep the elder "at home" or, at least, in a community setting. As a consequence, we have seen an expansion of the number and kinds of services that are delivered to elders in their homes—some of which were once only characteristic of institutional or residential care settings (i.e., physical therapy, hospice, or skilled nursing care). In part, the goal of such community-based services is to provide for the needs of elders by using the least disruptive intervention. To some extent, this principle has also been used as the rationale for the educational programs and support groups that have been created for family caregivers. Some have suggested that society can indirectly help elders by providing support services to those family caregivers who are already providing the bulk of long term care to elders (Springer and Brubaker, 1984).

By providing back-up and support to these informal helping systems, it has been argued that the needs of elders can be served in a more *natural,* or parsimonious, manner (Pancoast and Chapman, 1982).

Clarification of Perceptions, Expectations and Roles

Yet another principle important to working with families is that of clarifying the perceptions, expectations, and roles of client system constituents. A priori formulas for intervening in situations which involve the interactions of groups of people do not exist. Moreover, assumptions cannot validly be made that each individual involved, or potentially involved, perceives in the same way the objective and subjective realities of the situation being addressed. As a consequence, activities which tend to clarify differing perceptions must be undertaken (e.g., asking each member of the group to summarize his or her understanding of the care plan and to describe what is expected of each member or asking each member to summarize his or her understanding of the roles assigned to each other member).

The professional helper needs to be aware of potentially different perceptions at each step of the process of assisting the family. A common language must be developed to serve as a basis for communication among the family, and the terms of this language must be tested and re-tested to maximize effective communication (Devore and Schlesinger, 1987). Yet, the professional helper must also recognize that a high probability of miscommunication, misperception, or selective attending and understanding may continue to exist and must be taken into account when creating a care plan.

This potential for miscommunication and misperception may be particularly germane in the context of later life families. Faced with the escalating needs of an older parent, a son may find that old rivalries or jealousies will resurface among his siblings and may inhibit his ability to cope with the current crisis. Or, it may be that a woman is torn between the conflicting expectations for her as a ''daughter,'' a ''wife,'' and a ''mother'' and, as a result may feel pulled and torn between competing demands. Because the norms for caring for elderly family members may be changing in our society and given the most common caregiving relationships (i.e., spouse-to-spouse or adult child-to-parent) are so frequently emotionally charged and fraught with history, it is not surprising that the need for clarification is so keen (Springer and Brubaker, 1984; Cicirelli, 1983; Steinmetz and Amsden, 1983).

Expectations on the part of different members of the family system appear to be particularly subject to the pitfalls of the lack of clarity in communicating alluded to previously. The seasoned helping professional is, of course, aware of this possibility and its associated high probability, attempts to prevent it, but also is prepared to address it when it occurs. The ideal case would be one in which every member of the family understood the situation, understood what was expected of them, and understood the elements of the roles they were expected to perform. The reality is often much different and it is in these latter situations that the skills of a professional helper can enhance the effectiveness of a planned intervention. Contingencies need to be anticipated and alternative courses of action planned. Changes in care plans that result from fluctuations in the capacities of the social support networks that surround elders, however, should be seen as normal and expected and not necessarily as an indication of a failed plan of action or of professional incompetence.

Levels of Participation

In general, when determining who should be involved in a set of interventions on behalf of a client, practitioners should err on the side of "casting the net" widely and inviting the full participation of family members. Those who are going to contribute actively will do so, while those who will not participate, for whatever reason, aren't going to do so. Consistent with our earlier comments about the continuous nature of assessment, practitioners will become aware of the strengths and weaknesses of a family system as interactions proceed.

The helping professional needs to be aware, however, that the participation of all family members may very well *not* be achieved and that such a situation is neither unusual nor, necessarily, reflective of professional incompetence. Rather than zealously pursuing uniform levels of participation throughout a family, the interests of everyone are better served by recognizing that limitations in motivation, opportunity, and capacity, *do* exist. Indeed, family members should be assisted in understanding that differing levels should be permitted and accepted.

Within the context of later life families, practitioners must be careful not to make predeterminations about who will be, or should be, involved in family networking. This can be particularly dangerous in gender stereotyping. For example, it has long been a tenet of social gerontologists that adult daughters are more involved in the care of their parents than are sons (Brody, 1985). But, recent work has challenged the validity, and generalizability, of such assumptions (Coward, 1987). For our purses here, we would argue that it would be a mistake to assume that sons are not willing to be active participants in the care of their parents. Rather, we would suggest that it is advisable to provide opportunity and information to a wide network of family members and to allow those who are prepared to participate to do so.

However, it may be equally erroneous to build a care plan that is predicated on the equal distribution of responsibilities throughout a family. Some would have us believe, for example, that an elder who had three adult children had an advantage over an elder who had only one child. In reality, some recent research has indicated that later life families tend to have a "helping" child—no matter how many children are actually in the family (Hooyman and Lustbader, 1986). That is, in many later life families it appears that one of the children seems to take on the role of the "primary" helper and, in those situations, other siblings become supplements to the aid provided by that one person. It is as if there were a "queuing up" of helpers—one taking his or her turn now while the others wait in reserve. In families where this arrangement is dysfunctional (e.g., either because it is not meeting the needs of the elder or because it is resulting in resentment among siblings over the unequal distribution of caregiving tasks), it may be necessary for the professional helper to clarify the levels of participation of various family members and, if necessary, encourage shifts in responsibilities that bring about more equitable distributions.

The acceptance of diverse levels of commitment may also be necessary within the context of family decision-making. Unanimity among family members is difficult to achieve; and, of perhaps greater importance, it is quite often not essential to the resolution of the problem situation. The fervid pursuit of unanimity, therefore, should not be a goal in and of itself. Rather, it should be seen as positive if it can be achieved, but equally acceptable, and not reflective of professional incompetence, if it cannot be.

Use of Professional Authority

The professional helper is almost universally, by definition, assigned a superordinate position relative to his or her clients. Without certifying the merits or validity of this assignment, we can suggest that from this position the professional helper can derive a kind of power to be used to the benefit of the client. While members of the family may perceive unspoken expectations relative to the problem situation at hand, the professional helper is in a position either to reinforce those perceptions or, effectively, to "grant permission" to family members to act, think, or feel in a certain way. The skilled use of this "power" by a practitioner can facilitate family interactions on behalf of an identified client.

The adult son who lives out of state, for example, may be unable to drive his mother to the physician's office every other Tuesday to have her blood sugar checked—a chore that falls to his sister who lives in the same town as their mother. But, a professional helper may be able to alleviate the son's guilt, and/or the daughter's anger, by negotiating other tasks that the absent son can do for his mother (e.g., paying bills, filing out insurance reimbursement forms, tending to legal or banking records). All family members don't have to share equally in caregiving; rather, there needs to be an equitable distribution of the tasks according to the ability and circumstances of the family member to provide care. A third-party mediator, such as an agency social worker, can be useful and supportive to the family in the process of defining and identifying an equitable distribution of responsibilities.

CONCLUDING COMMENTS

In summary, the professional helper who works within the framework of the family needs to be aware of the overarching importance of continuing assessment, communication needs, the rights of the client and his or her significant others, the need for clarification of expectations and roles, and the limitations that are inherent in a family system. These limitations need not be seen as compromising the potential effectiveness of a proposed intervention but, rather, as realities which must be addressed. Further, the authority often granted a professional helper can be a means of facilitating family interaction through implied permission-granting and the selective reinforcement of feelings, actions, and cognitions on the part of family members. Awareness of self, professional roles, professional authority, and the processes of family intervention on the part of practitioners can be critical to forging collaborative partnerships between formal and informal helpers that serve to enhance the lives of older Americans.

REFERENCES

Biegel, D.E., Shore, B.K. and Gordon, E. (1984) *Building Support Networks for the Elderly: Theory and Applications*. Beverly Hills, California: Sage Publications, Inc.

Brandt, K., Hall, G., Pollitz-Hall, P., Lee, M.K., Martin, K. and Service, L. (1982) *Components of a Community-Based Long Term Care System for the Elderly* (Unit II). Iowa City: University of Iowa, Iowa Gerontology Model Project.

Brody, E.M. (1985) Parent care as a normative family stress. *The Gerontologist*, 25, 19-29.

Brown, K.B. and Drake, A.M. (1980) *Comparative Approaches to the Provision of Case Coordination Services*. Olympia: Washington Department of Social and Health Services, Office of Research.

Brubaker, T.H. (1985) Responsibility for household tasks: a look at golden anniversary couples aged 75 years and older. In W.A. Peterson and J. Quadagno (Eds.), *Social Bonds in Later Life; Aging and Interdependence*. Beverly Hills, California: Sage Publications.

Callahan, J.J., Jr. (1980) Responsibilities of families for their severely disabled elders. *Health Care Financing Review*, 1(3), 29-48.

Center for the Study of Social Policy. (1982) *Case Management in Long Term Care Programs*. Washington, D.C.: Author.

Cicirelli, V.G. (1983) Adult children and their elderly parents. In T.H. Brubaker (Ed.), *Family Relationships in Later Life*. Beverly Hills, California: Sage Publications.

Compton, B. and Galaway, B. (1984) *Social Work Processes*. Chicago: The Dorsey Press.

Coward, R.T. (1987) Factors associated with the configuration of the helping networks of noninstitutionalized elders. *Journal of Gerontological Social Work*, 10, 113-132.

Depner, C. and Ingersoll, B. (1980) Social support in the family context. Paper presented at the Thirty-third Annual Meeting of the Gerontological Society of America, San Diego, California, November.

Devore, W. and Schlesinger, E.G. (1987) *Ethnic-Sensitive Social Work Practice*. Columbus, Ohio: Merrill Publishing Company.

Graham, K.M. (1984) Developing family-centered aging services: orienting a rural community (Grant #90-AM-0041). Lewistown, Pennsylvania: Miffling-Juniata Area Agency on Aging, Inc.

Hartman, A. and Laird, J. (1983) *Family-Centered Social Work Practice*. New York: The Free Press.

Hess, B. and Soldo, B. (1985) Husband and wife networks. In W.J. Sauer and R.T. Coward (Eds.), *Social Support Networks and the Care of the Elderly: Theory, Research and Practice* (pp. 67-92). New York: Springer Publishing Company.

Hooyman, N. and Lustbader, W. (1986) *Taking Care: Supporting Older People and Their Families*. New York: The Free Press.

Horsley, D.L. (1985) Coordinated services in Vermont. Waterbury: Vermont Agency of Human Services.

Horsley, D.L., Fried, P. and Boice, M.R. (1980) Comparative analysis of four state aging networks: Arkansas, Pennsylvania, Utah, and Washington State (Grant #90-A-1618[01]). Silver Spring, Maryland: The Assistance Group for Human Resources Development.

Litwak, E. (1965) Extended kin relations in an industrial democratic society. In E. Shanas and G. Streib (Eds.), *Social Structures and the Family: Generational Relations*. (pp. 112-140). Englewood Cliffs, New Jersey: Prentice-Hall.

Loewenberg, F.M. (1983) *Fundamentals of Social Work Intervention: Basic Concepts, Intervention Activities and Core Skills*. New York: Columbia University Press.

Pancoast, D.L. and Chapman, N.J. (1982) Roles for informal helpers in the delivery of human services. In D. Biegel and A. Naparstek (Eds.), *Community Support Systems and Mental Health: Practice Policy and Research*. (pp. 234-271). New York: Springer Publishing Company.

Pincus, A. and Minahan, A. (1973) *Social Work Practice: Model and Method*. Itasca, Illinois: F. E. Peacock Publishers, Inc.

Sager, A. (1982) Living at home: the roles of public and informal supports in sustaining disabled older Americans (Grant #90-A-1679). Boston: Boston University, School of Public Health.

Sauer, W.J. and Coward, R.T. (Eds.) (1985) *Social Support Networks and the Care of the Elderly: Theory, Research and Practice*. New York: Springer Publishing Company.

Soldo, B.J. and Myllyluoma, J. (1983). Caregivers who live with dependent elderly. *The Gerontologist*, 23, 605-618.

Springer, D. and Brubaker, T.H. (1984) *Family Caregivers and Dependent Elderly*. Beverly Hills, California: Sage Publications.

Steinberg, R.M. and Jurkiewicz, V.C. (1980) A national director of case coordination programs for the elderly, with findings from the national survey (Grant #90-A-1280). Los Angeles: University of Southern California, Andrus Gerontology Center.

Steinmetz, S.K. and Amsden, D.J. (1983) Dependent elders, family stress, and abuse. In T.H. Brubaker (Ed.), *Family Relationships in Later Life*. Beverly Hills, California: Sage Publications.

Stephens, S.A. and Christianson, J.B. (1986) *Informal Care of the Elderly*. Lexington, Massachusetts: Lexington Books.

Stoller, E.P. and Earl, L.L. (1983) Help with activities of everyday life: Source of support for the noninstitutionalized elderly. *The Gerontologist*, 23, 64-70.

Strong, C. (1981) Families as caretakers of the elderly: a comparison of rural Indian and White families (Grant #90-AR-2076). Bellingham, Washington: Whatcom Counseling Clinic.

Thornton, C. and Dunston, S.M. (1986) Analysis of the benefits and costs of channeling: the evaluation of the national long term care demonstration (Contract #HHS-100-80-0157). Princeton: Mathematica Policy Research.

Van Nostrand, J. (1984, November) Population: Demography and Projections. In Primer Session, American Public Health Association/Veterans' Administration Invitational Conference on Long Term Care, Washington, D.C.

Wood, J.B. and Estes, C.L. (1985) Private non-profit organizations and community-based long term care. In C. Harrington, R.J. Newcomer, C.L. Estes and Associates (Eds.), *Long Term Care of the Elderly: Public Policy Issues*. Beverly Hills, California: Sage Publications.

Psychotherapy with the Elderly: A Systemic Model

James F. Keller
Mark C. Bromley

SUMMARY. The authors briefly review the contextual nature of the common problems faced by the elderly person that may require psychotherapy. An overview of traditional models for psychotherapy with the elderly is included. A systemic approach to psychotherapy with the elderly is highlighted, offering the practitioner several goals for the process of psychotherapy. Five strategies are presented for use in family therapy with older adults. The article concludes with an illustrative case study.

INTRODUCTION

In spite of major demographic and cultural shifts which support and empower the elderly, strong resistance remains regarding the efficacy and wisdom of psychotherapy for the elderly. "Put your energy and resources into therapy with the young," we are told. "You cannot teach an old dog new tricks" rumbles out of the mouths of a number of persons, surprisingly from many elderly themselves. By virtue of experience and accumulated wisdom the elderly have historically been looked to as the "bestowers of direction," the repositories of knowledge, that is, until today. In this age of information explosion change comes so rapidly as to nullify many of the benefits of accumulated knowledge. When the young become the counselors of the old we have experienced a kind of

James F. Keller, PhD, is affiliated with the Center for Family Services, Virginia Polytechnic Institute & State University, Blacksburg, VA 24061-0515. Mark C. Bromley, MS, is affiliated with the Center for Family Services, Virginia Polytechnic Institute & State University.

paradigm shift in which the teachers must teach without any traditions to inform and guide the teachers (Butler, 1975). Without a history of theory and practice of psychotherapy with the elderly, it is critical that the models proposed be grounded in an understanding of the elderly individual in context.

PROBLEMS OF THE ELDERLY

A systemic approach to the problems of the elderly is based on the assumption that the context of the older person is critical to understanding the special circumstances, needs, and problems of the elderly. Psychiatric problems with elderly persons tend to develop when their equilibrium is upset by stress that surpasses tolerable limits for the individual (Myers, 1982). The older adult as an adult in any other age-stage, is confronted with physical and situational changes that require personal adjustment and adaptability. For Myers, the goal of helping the older person to become integrated and comfortable in his/her familiar surroundings is possible given the recognition that problems are not a result of aging alone. When problems of the elderly are believed to be a result of aging alone, it is likely that common societal myths are contributing to that view. These myths constitute a major problem in psychotherapy with older persons. Edinberg (1985) presents support for seven common myths about the elderly: unproductivity; inevitable and irreversible loss of mental ability (senility), sexuality, and capacity for change; emotional fragility; inability to take care of themselves. Viewing all elderly as alike is a common mistake that disregards their variability of experiences, situations, and expectations. Families may overreact with their elder family members and depreciate their self-worth unwittingly as they act from these false beliefs. Also, the professional counselor or psychotherapist is not exempt from the negative impact of these myths.

A second major problem of the elderly is seen in the interaction of their physiological processes and their psychological well-being. Edinberg (1985) highlights various physical changes in the major body systems of the older person (e.g., physical discomfort from the musculoskeletal system, gastrointestinal problems, cardiopulmonary difficulties, changes in endocrine, reproductive and sensory systems) that may suggest psychological variations in the older adult population. In general, physical changes are best described as declining functions for older adults with most daily activities only being affected in times of stress (Edinberg, 1985). Declines from age will be different given a person's genetic makeup and their history of illnesses and the behavioral sequences that have developed around these physical problems. Physical changes due to the aging process or illness provide a context for the social and family interactions which frequently are perceived to be problematic to the older person or their family.

The third major problem for older adults that may prompt the need for psychotherapeutic services is the area of social and family interactions. Changes in social and family roles, retirement, illness, death of friends, loss of a spouse, often are interpreted as having negative implications by elderly individuals and their families and may have the effect of changing living arrangements and diminishing independence. Brody (1986) concludes that whenever the need arises for adult children to involve themselves in the care of their parent a central issue is the tension between dependence and independence. More elderly widows are living alone (women as head of household in 1940 was 40%; in 1977 was 49.6%) while elderly men tend to either live alone or remarry (Mindel, 1986). Intergenerational living arrangements are potentially difficult as issues of control, authority, and responsibility are encountered daily.

Retirement can be a controversial life-cycle issue for older adults. The adaptation to the loss of the prescribed social role that was provided by the work place, the economic impact of the transition and/or a possible relocation can be important to the well-being of the elder and his/her children (Edinberg, 1985; Myers, 1982). The potential for marital conflict is known to increase at this stage. Feelings of decreased personal freedom of wives and "suffocation" from the husband's increased presence can be a problem. Other issues frequently noted include: strain related to wives' perceived attempts at organizing the husbands' time and their dislike of this outside control; the division of household labor (Troll, 1986).

As chronically ill or impaired older adults need care, difficulties are likely to increase in their relationship. For those who can afford it, such care is often given with the use of paid helpers to assist in difficult tasks. Spousal care has its limits, especially with increased age (Cantor, 1986) due to age-related needs and predisposition to poor health. Adult children were the next greatest source of care, second only to spouses (Shanas, 1986; Cantor, 1986). Such caregivers are predominantly married women with families who experience personal and financial stress from their own middle-age life pursuits i.e., employment, raising children, and maintaining separate households. Considerable intergenerational stress derives from these developments and may or may not be recognized by the family members as an important focus of family psychotherapy. The patterns of interaction that surround and weave through the overall context of the elderly are vital for psychotherapy. The number of contributors to models of psychotherapy with the elderly remain small. As the population of aging members increases, interest will no doubt increase.

MAJOR CONTRIBUTORS

Edinberg (1985) presents several approaches in the treatment of the elderly. Psychoanalytic therapists assume that pathology is rooted in the unconscious conflicts of the past and that insight can be achieved through review and interpretation of individual and family history. Behavioral and cognitive approaches focus on overt behavior and thought processes. The behavioral therapist may use relaxation, systematic desensitization, or reinforcement techniques while a cognitive therapist would address irrational thought patterns and inappropriate problem solving methods that are used by the elder. A third model makes use of humanistic and creative-expressive modalities. These focus on the present experience of the older adult and the exploration of their subjective context to highlight conflicts in their current life. Humanistic approaches aim for optimal development of the individual as a result of increasing the client's awareness. Creative-expressive therapy may use music, art, or dance in eliciting feelings and may provide socialization as a secondary benefit for the elderly person.

A fourth model is the family therapy approach. Family therapy differs from other modalities by its assumption that the family patterns are the source of the dysfunction and the needed focus of intervention. Consequently, the older adult's current social and relational context receives attention as well as the perceived ineffective behavioral patterns between generations of families.

Herr and Weakland (1979) developed a systematic approach to psychotherapy with the elderly and their families through their practice at the Mental Research Institute. The approach is based on three major assumptions:

1. The focus is on the here-and-now situation and is thereby accessible to the therapist, the elder, and the family for observation, evaluation, and influence.
2. The "handling" of problems by the parties involved is viewed as a more significant focus than the problem itself. The behaviors that occur around a problem and the evaluation of the problem are of primary importance in this model.
3. An emphasis of this approach is on small but strategic changes that will become part of the family system's interaction. This means therapy is brief and should be more attractive to health care providers than long-term psychotherapy.

Keller and Hughston (1981) presented a systemic therapy model which views the elderly as living within a system that includes the social context, interaction with that context, and feedback processes that are operative within the context of interactions. The assumptions behind their model include:

1. Interrelationships are of primary importance in the client's daily social exchanges.
2. Idiosyncratic personality traits of the elderly were developed from their perceptions of the context of their family of origin and their individual choices in response to that context. In a continuing and widening system these patterns now contribute to the shaping of sequences of behavior in the family of procreation.
3. Behavior in the present is of primary concern although past behavior may be important in providing points of comparison and illumination of current behavior.

Recently, Viney and associates (1986) have proposed a model for the psychosocial functioning in the elderly which focuses on the individual's personal constructs and/or the family construct system that the family holds. The therapeutic relationship addresses constructs that are too loose and have little predictive ability for the future or are too tight and do not allow free exploration of possibilities. Reconstruing by the client is seen as the client escaping from, modifying, or being more active in their personal/family constructs. The theoretical emphases of family models have enabled practitioners to attend to the present relevance of problems, the interaction of individuals and the meaning of the situation an elderly individual may be experiencing. This perspective has important implications for the goals of therapeutic interventions with the elderly.

PSYCHOTHERAPY PROCESS GOALS WITH THE ELDERLY

The context of psychotherapy with the elderly would presume a general support system addressing such issues as income, diet, health, health care resources, housing and transportation. Although the purpose of this discussion is a more focused presentation of psychotherapy processes with the elderly, a supportive network of professionals is a significant resource for broad systemic needs. Referrals for concurrent medical evaluations for example, may bring important data to the psychotherapy context. The specific goals of psychotherapy with older persons should include at least the following:

1. It is important to have the whole family present for therapy. The context of a systems' paradigm for working with the elderly assumes the presenting symptomatic behavior is best understood and treated as a part of family patterns. While specific individual behaviors or physical conditions may begin presumably outside interactions with family members, inevitably the family (whether near or far away) will react to these behaviors or conditions. These responses to the problem become patterned, recursive and are repeated within family transactions. However, members frequently frame "the problem" as lodged *within* one or several elderly family

members. Actually the "individual problem" which triggered the symptomatic pattern may or may not have long since been dealt with, but the associated patterned interactional behaviors shaped over time remain. Elderly live within social contexts, give and receive responses which shape the behavior of others. The responses of family members are seen as completing loops which shape the older person's responses in continuing recursive feedback loops. These feedback loops develop into repeated patterns which frequently mask as individual problems.

Since an initial task of psychotherapy is to help the family identify its purpose for seeking therapy, it is assumed that the most helpful therapeutic context for work with the elderly is to have the whole family present. Having access to direct observation of family patterns is considerably superior to one individual's skewed interpretation. Family members are typically more cooperative about traveling in for the session than may be perceived by the elderly person(s). Having 2-3 hour sessions can accommodate family members coming in from distant locations, and are potentially more productive than several one hour sessions.

2. The initial goals of psychotherapy with the family include a significant emphasis on joining socially and therapeutically with them as a group. This process should not be shortened in order to "get on with therapy." It is therapy! Care should be taken to give respect to the elderly family members, at the same time giving recognition to the children as adults. The goal is to give the parents respect and position without re-introducing their control; to identify the children as children without infantasizing them. If this is effective the elderly will begin to feel less like they are pathological, that they have a place in the family and the other family members will not feel singled out for blame controlled by a coalition of parents and therapist. This stage should *not* be understood as an event once having been accomplished requires no return. Social and therapeutic joining will occur again and again throughout the therapy process. An important element of "therapeutic joining" involves helping the family clarify, as specifically as possible, their goals for therapy. These may or may not be obvious at the beginning of the session and can be raised later in the session(s).

Having the family identify/clarify its goals for therapy is important for several reasons: (1) It is not the therapist, but they, and they alone who know their own family's needs/desires; (2) it is not the therapist, but they who will live with and continue to be affected by whatever changes occur in the session; (3) each family is uniquely different and consequently, few, if any, universal prescriptions exist which can be applied to all. The family may attempt to enroll the therapist as the expert for them, and/or the therapist may feel more helpless if he/she is not the "healer." To succumb to this seduction may have the appearance of short-term benefits, but in the short and long haul subverts the family's resources.

3. A basic assumption of this model is that families are essentially healthy, i.e., that persons make the best choices they can, given the resources they possess. It is assumed that the family, including the elderly, have resources for changing or coping with their patterned responses. The role of the therapist is one of identifying these strengths and encouraging behaviors that result in their release. A very popular Western assumption, however, is that to be elderly is to be dependent, inactive, protected from risk and responsibility. It should not surprise anyone when this expectation is all too often fulfilled. A further complicating contextual influence is the historical tradition in psychotherapy of focusing on pathology. Identifying individual and family deficits is still seen by many as an essential component for getting to the "helping" process. The therapeutic microscope too frequently focuses on psychological disorders. Unfortunately, labeling deviance appears to contribute more to the needs of the therapist than the older person. A diagnostic pigeon-hole may add another significant layer of emotional and psychological stress to the individual. Pathology seems better understood as a product of the human mind, generated by our own realities. To presume that our concepts are synonymous with reality is like confusing a map of a region with the region. A diagnosis cannot be the reality, but represents the therapist's projected view of reality. Diagnosis can be a useful way of describing if we remain aware that we created the concept. A problem for many when working with the elderly occurs when things are not the way the therapist wants them to be or thinks they should be. Unfortunately then, there is a strong temptation to label the person as pathological.

Learning how to identify strengths in the elderly and their families requires a different way of thinking about psychotherapy. Scanning clients for their strengths will be facilitated by the therapist's identification and acceptance of his/her strengths and comfort with their expression. When the therapist searches for points of strength in clients, areas of incompetence recede and competence is allowed to come to the fore. An added advantage of this approach is that the client does not have to deal with the additional burden that pathology descriptions impart. Further, if an approach that emphasizes understanding and treating *patterns of behavior* is used, scapegoating individuals is not essential.

4. From various physiological and environmental sources individual stresses can erupt. Persons in the near and far environment respond to these stresses with some degree of support, criticism, indifference, worry. Most adult children's responses contain some or all of the above, flavored usually by a mind-set which assumes that the elderly are fragile and need to be relieved of responsibilities. This stance reflects a kind of reversal of the developmental growth process framing the elder as a "child." A major therapeutic goal is one which emphasizes the resources of the elderly for independence and avoids "caring too much" for them. "Caring too much" is defined as doing things for them which they could be doing for themselves. The therapist's goal should be guided by acting in behalf of their "growth." The therapist will want to be alert to transactions that occur in the session which support or hinder the growth of family members.

5. An important therapeutic goal is the identification of needs, responsibilities, and expectations of all family members, with particular attention given to the elderly. As a family passes through the various developmental stages, expectations of its family members change. This is not a problem in itself. Problems may occur because the family seldom talks about what has happened. Frustration and disappointments accrue and patterned responses begin to develop. The family feedback system around these developments continues with "the problem" getting increasingly deposited with the elderly. An important therapeutic goal involves identifying these patterns and clarifying the goals and expectations of family members.

6. Creating a context that encourages an awareness of underlying "behavioral-beliefs" is an additional goal of psychotherapy with

the elderly. Conscious or intentional "beliefs" are not the focus. Rather, at issue are those more or less unconscious convictions about oneself, family, friends that can be identified only by inference from tracking patterns of behavior. For example, a couple, both in their mid-seventies, experienced a recurring problem involving the wife regularly calling the eldest daughter discussing the depressed and withdrawing behaviors of the elderly husband. The wife and daughter resisted bringing the entire family in to therapy, saying it would further alienate and depress father. After agreeing to bring the entire family to the sessions the therapist tracked the underlying belief represented in the behavior of the mother and adult daughter. The identified behavioral beliefs were: women are inherently stronger emotionally than men, men are fragile emotionally, and should be protected. If the elderly male in this case had been seen by himself for treatment, the therapist could unwittingly have contributed to this covert family belief. By bringing in the father, involving him in the family's communication circuits, new family strengths and patterns around these assets were begun.

7. Finally, an important goal of psychotherapy with the elderly involves the development of adaptation options. Once the family's goals for therapy have been established, with individual and family needs and expectations identified, the stage is set for creating adaptation options that fit individual's and the family's goals. These goals presume the elderly continue to have some measure of resources and strength, that the family is ready not only to allow but to encourage the elderly to function independently to the maximum of their abilities, that support is to be defined as doing for the elderly that which they cannot do for themselves. Strategies and techniques for achieving these goals will be discussed in the following section.

STRATEGIES OF PSYCHOTHERAPY
WITH OLDER PERSONS

A basic assumption regarding strategies of psychotherapy with any age group is it appears that they cannot be directly taught. The importance of this generalization is not based on the complexity of psychotherapy nor does the issue revolve around the debate of whether psychotherapy is an art or a set of techniques. The question has more to do with the assumption that every individual is unique, every therapist owns a different set of biological, cultural, social, and familial experiences, possesses cognitive and emotional filters that are individually idiosyncratic to him/her. Each individual's make-up determines what will be perceived and experienced. Individuals only "know" what their own internal system tells them about what is going on. Individuals and families can be perturbed by confronting different individuals' perceptions of reality. How the individual perceives this different perception of reality, whether the reader or the person in therapy, will depend on how he/she defines the confrontation. In a psychotherapeutic context each individual creates his/her own reality. At the same time persons consensually agree about certain commonly interpreted experiences, i.e., define their "family reality." Family members in therapy will screen communicational content (both covert and overt) through their own filters as they continuously frame and reframe their own realities. Therapists reading this material will do the same. There is no way a pure and unadulterated "reality" can be transferred, intact (i.e., as it is presumed to be in the purveyer's reality), from the written page to the reader's reality nor from a therapist to a family or family member. There is every likelihood that the reader of these pages will filter what is written here in uniquely individual ways with no two readers having completely matching interpretations. It is no different in therapy. It is not so much that this assumption changes the nature of psychotherapy, but rather that this view offers a different choreography. Therapy cannot be seen as a type of "objective" content that can be given like a medical prescription which "corrects," "reshapes" problematic symptoms, i.e., "cures" the individual or family. It can be seen as the presenting of other "realities," other options to the individual/family. What they do when "perturbed" by these realities, the reality they create from "bumping up against" these new realities, belongs to the family/elderly individual. This is a most exciting aspect, a revolutionary position for psychotherapy in which even the form of therapy is constructive and hopeful.

The following are a list of primary strategies and techniques for presenting options with the elderly. The list is not meant to be exhaustive nor all of them useful with everyone, or every presenting problem.

1. Emotional Connections Review: When the complaint revolves around too much family closeness, too much protection, i.e., emotional fusion, a "family meeting" may be suggested. At the meeting the therapist might meet individually (with the elder) for several sessions to identify the particular issues which appear, from his/her perspective, to be useful as an agenda for the "family meeting." Of particular interest would be emotionally unsatisfying patterns of behavior involving the elder and other family members. After identifying the primary concerns of over-protection, for example, details of typical behavioral patterns and emotional connections can be pursued, from the elder's perspective. It is usually helpful to go over various options for the elder in communicating these issues to the whole family. In most circumstances it is better for the elder to assume responsibility for initiating the concerns to the family group.

2. Techniques for the Family Group Meeting: Initially, it is of paramount importance to socially join with the family. This technique may be of continued usefulness at various times throughout the session(s). Joining at an emotional level represents still another level of identification with the family. This involves a genuine attempt by the therapist to feel with the family their discomfort, a listening to the therapist's own internal responses to the family and an observation of the behavioral patterns reflected in the "new system": family and therapist. Awareness of the therapist's view of the new system's behavioral patterns will give him/her a point of emotional contact with the family and provide a counterpoint for understanding and joining the elder's perspective of the family.

Other strategies for the family group meeting include the structuring of the transition to the elder's data from the Emotional Connections Review. Observing the family communication tracks and waiting for a more "natural" point of entry is usually desirable. Encouraging the elder without taking responsibility for the communication is a tricky task to which the therapist should be especially attentive. When the issues at hand involve the elder and a particular family member, communication can be facilitated by arranging the seating in ways that make more direct communication and eye contact likely. Seating arrangements which encourage appropriate hierarchies and emotional connections should be considered, e.g., helping an elder female to change seats to bring her next to her husband and out of the middle of a seating arrangement flanked by the children.

The process of asking the family questions, on the order of the Milan model of "neutral questioning" (Selvini, Boxcolo, Cecchin, & Prata, 1980; Tomm, 1987), helps the family to come to grips with their multiple perspectives of the family dynamics. The therapist who understands the principles of neutral questioning but lacks experience, could try a more basic two step process: (1) identify your own hypotheses about the family patterns; (2) instead of directly informing the family of your hypotheses, select a hypothesis and ask questions as a way of testing it and allowing the family to think about the hypothesis at the same time.

3. Probe for Strengths: Until relatively recently the elderly in our history have been the most potent of all age groups in terms of knowledge, power, and influence. Today's knowledge explosion has all but reversed that standing. The effect on the elderly has been to render them increasingly impotent members of society. As repositories of information, there is little likelihood that the elderly will ever return to prominence and power (to the extent that information brings power). However, as repositories of emotional connections, their beginnings and historical nurturance, the elderly are significant resources of value to the family. There is no better resource for the adult children to probe for the processes of transmission of anxiety and patterns of solution practiced across generations. Operating from the assumptions of this approach the therapist is guided by this fundamental maxim: probe for strengths, seek positive family resources. Search for recognized as well as unacknowledged strengths. Acquaint the family with these treasures through the medium of questions, i.e., follow the steps in 2 preceding.

4. Therapy as a World of Counterpointing Realities: Many families who present for therapy presume it to be a process of finding the "right" solution to a particular problem. If it is impossible to impart a "right" solution, intact, then therapy need not burden itself with unrealizable expectations. What appears to be appropriate is to unfold to the family the many "realities" represented by all the

members. No one person's reality is understood to be "the reality" and all are viable interpretations of the "life of the family in question." Introducing the family to a "world of counterpointing realities" is a significant therapeutic intervention. The acceptance of this assumption requires a respect for the various counterpointing realities, which in turn means more respect for the purveyor of each reality. To the extent that the family functions from a world of counterpointing realities, new behavioral patterns and emotional connections are going to evolve. Acceptance of this assumption makes genuine communication all the more important. Consensual agreement becomes a priority to move the family beyond the impasse of counterpointing realities. This requires compromise and the development of new behavioral patterns and emotional connections in the system.

Strategically, the therapist will present not only the family's realities, but can seek, through questioning to clarify, to challenge, and to push for expansion of the "realities" of the members. This process allows the family to filter, alter, and amend the therapist's "realities" as well as those of other members. Allowing the family to decide whether and how to change family patterns and emotional connections is a fundamental goal of therapy, not finding a "right" solution to a family problem. Changing the practiced patterns and emotional connections allows the family to change its "realities." Changing "realities" opens new and creative resources for problem solution by the family.

5. Structured reminiscence involves the recalling of past facts or experiences to conscious awareness, a useful intervention with some depressed elderly patients (Keller & Hughston, 1981). Discussing the many and varied life experiences from the frame of "counterpointing realities" allows the possibility for amending/filtering of the particular "reality-frame" of the memories by the elder.

Many elderly individuals live with losses and need help in constructive grieving. Reminiscence is a useful adaptation strategy for dealing with the emotional and psychological dislocation of grief, e.g., feelings of desertion, guilt, and emotional paralysis. An elderly man complained that he could not let himself enjoy experiences with friends and family members because his wife could no longer be present to share them. Recalling his life experiences with his wife, in some detail, allowed him to discover that his wife had, over the life of their marriage, indulged in many happy experiences with her friends and relatives which he had not shared. This "counterpoint reality" enabled him to separate him and his experiences from the memory of his wife. Reminiscence is a very important tool for psychotherapy with the elderly individual.

CASE EXAMPLE

An elderly female was referred by her family physician for psychotherapy. She had complained of depression, sleep difficulties and increased conflict with her husband. Generally the marriage had been a happy one, but now one with the husband somewhat out of place after a recent retirement from a very stressful management position. The couple had moved back to an area where they had lived earlier in their marriage. Friends and family members provided a generally happy social network. There did not seem to be any reason for being depressed so Mrs. C. assumed the problem was organic. Testing revealed no physical difficulties other than normal aging.

Mrs. C. presented for therapy with considerable evidence of depressive behavior. She described the context of her depression (from her reality) as generalized dissatisfaction with her life. She had come to believe something was wrong with her. The second session was given to a review of the patterns of behavior that she experienced with her husband and her two daughters. Special attention was paid to how depressive behaviors affected and were affected by family interactions. She indicated that her father had died shortly after he had retired and how this had crushed her mother. She remembered her mother as not being prepared to take on the responsibilities and decisions that independence forced on her. She saw her mother get increasingly depressed and remained so until she died two years later. At the time of her father's death, Mrs. C. was very busy with her two young daughters and a career. She remembered saying, "I just don't have time to grieve." The therapist's initial hypothesis was two-fold: (1) Mrs. C.'s unresolved grief for her parents was a contributor to the current stated problem in an as yet unknown systemic and individual manner; (2) Mr. C.

was able to postpone dealing with his retirement problem while Mrs. C.'s difficulty took such prominence. The therapist decided to examine the interactional nature of the problem first, and later deal with the individual aspects of the apparent unresolved grief. Mrs. C. was encouraged to bring her husband, her two daughters, and their husbands to the next session.

The family seated themselves with the daughters' husbands on the sofa, Mrs. C. in a single chair, the eldest daughter sitting next to her holding her hand and the other daughter and Mr. C. in two single chairs across the room from Mrs. C. Each family member's view of the "family reality" was requested. Everyone seemed to be puzzled by Mrs. C.'s depression but concluded that something needed to be "done for her." Her husband felt that the physician should prescribe medication immediately. Family patterns of response to Mrs. C.'s depressive behavior and communication were tracked. The husband and eldest daughter were asked to exchange seats. Mrs. C. was asked eventually about her feelings regarding her husband's retirement. She immediately began weeping. Mr. C. was encouraged to comfort her. She got worse. Mr. C. appeared embarrassed and sat back in his chair. The eldest daughter ran across the room to kneel beside her mother. As the family processed the transactions that had just occurred, Father stated that he felt that he did not know how to relate to his wife since they had retired. She seemed to him to be very distant. Mrs. C. described her fear of Mr. C.'s death upon his retirement, just like what her father had experienced. Mr. C. asked Mrs. C. why she had become so distant. She stated that she feared becoming more vulnerable if she allowed herself to get closer and then have him die. Recognizing this view of the family reality as viable, the therapist offered an additional counterpointing reality (through asking questions): Who was most and least affected by Mrs. C.'s depression and emotional withdrawal? How did her behavior affect the husband and his problem with retirement? Her view of herself? Her decisions about how to participate in retirement? What effect would a change from depression to a more general satisfaction with life have? On each family member? On husband and his retirement? On Mr. and Mrs. C.'s marriage? What hidden resources had the family been using as they struggled together? Each family member offered their realities, many counterpointing, some consensual. The therapist avoided the trap of depression as Mrs. C.'s problem and probed the family's strengths for resolution of their interactional issues. The task of the family was to come to some consensual agreement about their counterpointing realities. The couple faced this issue as well. The family was seen for a second time together, followed by a number of sessions with just the couple. Finally, Mrs. C. was seen by herself to work on remaining unresolved grief about her parents through reminiscence procedures. A summary session was held to involve Mr. C. in the developments of grief work that impacted him and the marriage.

As larger proportions of the population continue to "grey," psychotherapy with the elderly represents a critical and exciting new focus area. Assessment and treatment procedures that take advantage of family resources offer significant advantages for the field of psychotherapy.

REFERENCES

Brody, E.M. (1986). Parent care as a normative stress. In L.E. Troll (Ed.), *Family issues in current gerontology* (pp. 97-119). New York: Springer Publishing Company.

Butler, R.V. (1975). *Why survive: Being old in America*. New York: Harper & Row.

Cantor, M.H. (1986). Strain among caregivers: A study of experience in the United States. In L.E. Troll (Ed.), *Family issues in current gerontology* (pp. 246-263). New York: Springer.

Edinberg, M.A. (1985). *Mental health practice with the elderly*. Englewood Cliffs, NJ: Prentice-Hall.

Herr, J.J., & Weakland, J.H. (1979). *Counseling elders and their families*. New York: Springer.

Keller, J.F., & Hughston, G.A. (1981). *Counseling the elderly: A systems approach*. New York: Harper & Row.

Mindel, C.H. (1986). Multigenerational family households: Recent trends and implications for the future. In L.E. Troll (Ed.), *Family issues in current gerontology* (pp. 269-283). New York: Springer.

Myers, J.M. (1982). Psychiatric problems. In T.G. Duncan (Ed.), *Over 55: A handbook on health* (pp. 443-468). Philadelphia: The Franklin Institute Press.

Selvini, M.P., Boscolo, L., Cecchin, G., & Prata, G. (1980). Hypothesizing, circularity, neutrality: Three guidelines for the conductor of the session. *Family Process, 19*, 3-12.

Shanas, E. (1986). The family as a social support system in old age. In L.E. Troll (Ed.), *Family issues in current gerontology* (pp. 85-96). New York: Springer.

The Life Review:
An Underutilized Strategy
for Systemic Family Intervention

George A. Hughston
Nancy J. Cooledge

SUMMARY. This paper explores reflection upon the past and the potential it may hold for the systemic family practitioner. Reminiscence is viewed to be an underutilized and underinvestigated strategy for intervention with the elderly and their families. The paper includes a list of benefits for the therapist, as well as individuals and families involved in the counseling process. Systemic family therapy should make effective use of reflection upon past events in order to develop positive understanding of the complex role experience plays in avoidance of repeating past mistakes and the creation of future success.

Reminiscence technique is a strategy not commonly utilized in systemic family intervention. This paper examines the potential impact reminiscence may provide in family therapy with the elderly. By design, a brief review of research reveals conflicting and somewhat confusing scientific data concerning the effects of long term memory upon the elderly and their families. It should be noted that indeed there is a deficit of consistent evidence. But, a myriad of benefits stand to be gained from applying this technique in appropriate situations. Clearly, it is evident that reflection upon the past holds promise for those practitioners who utilize it properly.

George A. Hughston, PhD, is with the Department of Family Resources and Human Development, Arizona State University, Tempe, AZ 85287. Nancy J. Cooledge is with Segmented Markets, Inc., 7955 East Chaparral #15, Scottsdale, AZ 85253. Correspondence should be addressed to Dr. Hughston.

Theory without practical application is meaningless. Most reminiscence literature has come from theoreticians rather than practitioners, therefore contributing to a lack of congruent findings. Without congruent findings providing both positive and negative results of reminiscence, the transition is left to the practitioner's interpretations and therapeutic skills. In other words, what works for one may not work for another.

REVIEW OF THE LITERATURE

Utilization of past experiences is not a new idea to avoid unpleasant consequences associated with current behavior. During biblical times, people were encouraged to reflect upon their mistakes and not repeat prior errors. In other words, constructive use of past experiences was viewed as beneficial (Paul, 54-58 a.d.).

Only during the past twenty-five years, have. social science investigators revived interest in reminiscence. The work of Butler (1963) led the scientific community away from what had been a predominately negative view of the psychologically dysfunctional nature of past memory. Prior to his work, past memory had been thought to obscure awareness of present realities. Butler introduced the concept of the "Life Review" as a "naturally occurring universal mental process, characterized by the progressive return to consciousness of past experiences (p. 66)." For Butler, the life review allowed unresolved conflicts to be surveyed and reintegrated with positive outcomes. These outcomes included wisdom, serenity, and increased understanding of both personal and environmental nature. Although Butler noted the possibility of a negative life review triggering despair, fitful antagonisms and increased depression, he has purported that the benefits predominate.

McMahon and Rudick (1964) defined reminiscence as an act or habit of thinking about, or relating to, past experiences one considers most personally significant. Their research revealed positive correlation between amount of reminiscence and successful adaptation to old age. They noted reflection upon past experiences to be difficult and less frequent for subjects diagnosed as being clinically depressed.

Lewis (1971) emphasized the positive adaptive nature of reminiscence in his comparative self-concept investigation between those who reminisce and those who do not. Although Lewis' scores did not differ initially, with the inducement of stress those who reminisce were found to significantly increase their self-concept compared to those who did not. Lieberman and Falk (1971) viewed middle-aged subjects to use reminiscence in problem solving while elderly subjects utilized reminiscence to enhance personal life satisfaction. Aged people were found to use reminiscence in restructuring meaningful interpersonal relationships more than middle-aged people. It is also noted that Lieberman and Falk found reminiscence to be a significant influence upon those older people who faced stressful life situations such as impending change of residence.

Differences in oral and silent reminiscing were investigated by Havighurst and Glasser (1972) who measured both frequency and quality of reminiscence. Their research indicated high frequency of reminiscence was positively related to pleasant effects and effective personal-social adjustment.

Self-reports from Fallots (1980) revealed middle-age and older female subjects experienced a decrease in anxiety and depression following reminiscence. The Fallots' data conclude the major effect of reminiscence was reduction of negative mood rather than an increase in positive emotion. Further exploration regarding mood by Snyder and White (1982) found their subjects more prone to remember past events related to current mood state. The Snyder and White research indicated depressed people were more likely to focus upon negative past events. Retrieval of predominately positive or negative memories could be a previously overlooked measure of mood having therapeutic implications.

Reminiscence may be used in order to stimulate thinking processes in elderly people and may be associated in increases in thinking abilities (Hughston and Merriam, 1982). Research support for extensive programs using past memory suggests tremendous possibility for its utilization as an intervention technique with the elderly. Therapists involved with the aged and their families may find structured reminiscence programs of benefit (Keller and Hughston, 1981).

A review of data related to reflection upon the past indicates a lack of precision in ability to predict outcomes of a reminiscence experience. Therapists who choose to utilize techniques that maximize reflection upon the past should do so with knowledge of risk taking and respect for the unknown.

This brief summary of a portion of the research illustrates mixed results related to effects and potential therapeutic value of reflection upon the past.

The best practitioners are not necessarily benevolent eclectics, but rather remain capable of maintaining an eclectic tool box of therapeutic strategies and recognize the most appropriate tools for the uniqueness of the situation. Reminiscence should be one of their tools.

BENEFITS FOR SYSTEMIC FAMILY INTERVENTION

The initial establishment of rapport is of paramount necessity for effective family intervention. A therapist will benefit from quick and meaningful rapport created with the elderly client and family through utilization of recalling past experiences shared by the participants. Identification of topic areas of significance to a particular family will require substantial homework by the therapist. Following the intake interview, a goal is to maximize general areas that are unique to the particular family. For example, family experiences may be happily remembered and may provide an introduction to the underlying root of the problem.

Reminiscence is potentially therapeutic by nature of its historical perspective. Just as Texans revel in historical reflection upon the Alamo, so do families and individuals enjoy past successes. Careful examination of developmental aspects of family success and overcoming obstacles may serve as a point of departure for dealing successfully with present crisis. Past abilities to successfully resolve conflict is the foundation for present crisis resolution. Reminiscence may serve as the catalyst/monitor allowing a family to view both strengths and weaknesses from a learning perspective of benefit to the entire group.

A discussion of life-span successes may be absent of total accuracy. Still, general explanations may be utilized by the therapist to create a bridge from past to present. As Pear (quoted by Havighurst and Glasser, 1972, p. 246) wrote, "The mind never photographs. It paints pictures." All reminiscence will be subjective and distorted by one's perception. Value to the family practitioner is in no way diminished by lack of accuracy. Parents and children will view the same past event quite differently. For example, taking out the garbage may be reflected upon by adult children as a most unpleasant event dictated by a hysterical, tyrannical parent who was, "Unrelenting for household perfection." The elderly parent's reflection upon the same event would include such elements as a constant battle against offensive odor, ants, roaches and adolescent laziness.

Therapeutic potential from such conflicting recollections depends upon the skill of the counselor. Conflicting family recollections offer therapists opportunities to mediate, negotiate and recognize present family relationships. Although these experiences occurred many years ago, patterns of manipulation, control, power, affection and conflict resolution remain eternal without intervention of some type. A general assumption may be that the average parent is 700 years old unless some type of educational intervention has occurred.

Memories provide a basis for current problem resolution in order to launch both individuals and families toward fresh vantage points from where they may overlook, reevaluate and move on. Family reminiscence can help them recognize and break a chain of self-defeating behaviors. For many, repetitious mistakes appear to be a way of life. The same errors obvious to the therapists will be found in multiple generations. Sons and daughters repeat patterns of behaviors learned from parents and grandparents. In other words, fourth generational problems such as habitual unemployment, child abuse, incest, alcoholism, and other self-defeating behaviors may be characteristic of many family systems. Effective systemic family therapy utilizes positive reflection upon the past in order to break behavioral chains.

Social contacts based upon similar cohort experiences serve to validate and support self-esteem. Sharing similarities of experiences with others, i.e., survivors of the Batan Death March, provides opportunities to reexamine one's identity and reemphasize the importance of this experience to both the individual and family. A colorful legacy provides family congruence and identity. Although one elderly family member experienced this particular family event, a model of survival may be transferred to younger members. Reminiscence may have a profound impact upon the entire family and its sense of continuity, history, integrity and success.

Clinicians familiar with family history may structure reminiscence activities to stimulate memories of past events. Family history will be supplemented by the rich and colorful heritage every individual, couple and family contributes to the family system. Artifacts having a historical perspective such as photographs, music, furniture and even clothing may further link individuals to one another. Grandfather's World War I uniform, medals, and war souvenirs will contribute to meaningful cross-age group bonding regardless of differences in age or time. Similar emotions reside within each family member. Although these emotions may be expressed in many ways, reminiscence allows recognition of their existence, responsibility for their control and selective expression regardless of age.

Life review of events serve to orient even the most confused young person by promoting recognition that they are not the first to experience similar problems. In fact, the old do know more about being young than the young know about being old. The family therapist may capitalize upon these age differences through reflection of past quests. The grandfather who dropped out of school, ran away and joined the circus when he was 16, was not the first teenager or the last to leave, return, reintegrate and rebound to productive, responsible adulthood. Young people may benefit from therapeutic intervention emphasizing the realities that old people have successfully resolved encounters similar to theirs.

Older family members remain models of life's changeability, survivability and adaptability. Surviving and adapting to rapid change in a modern technological world may indeed be no more stressful than adapting to the trauma of an outdoor toilet during a cold winter night. Every family system requires adaptation to stress and change. Current stressors are no more traumatic than past stressful events. The young often attempt to overemphasize current trauma of a complex and perplexing society. Their plight is indeed no more traumatic that those previously, successfully resolved by their elders.

Toffler's classical *Future Shock* (1970) proposed bombardment by technology as responsible for many stress related difficulties. Reminiscence may provide examples of brutal reality versus mythological fantasies of stress. The older person will probably attest to the fact that there is equal or less stress involved in selecting meat, fish or poultry from a well stocked meat counter than having to catch and kill an unwilling, noncooperative chicken.

There are tremendous advantages to thoughtful counselor intervention directed toward involvement of the young through the reminiscence process. Within this context, logical ties will be formulated between the adolescent and the elderly. Both are in similar low power, low status positions revolving around the high power, high status of middle age. Reminiscence therapy may provide the skilled counselor opportunity to elicit similarities of status or power among family members.

Material stored and revised over a lifetime may provide interesting, innovative alternative strategies for younger people to effectively resolve crisis and stress. If the aged person has learned from his/her historical experiences, then accuracy in transferring problem solving techniques and skills to current 20th century problems is no illusion. The act or process of recalling the past (Butler, 1963, p. 66) should contain a prescription for problem and conflict resolution that is often overlooked by the practitioner.

Many grown children do not ask for or respect advice of their parents. Usually, the meddlesome older person is the last with whom to share problems. The reality is that they often barely tolerate each other. Under the guidance of the skilled therapist, family rapport may be established allowing two-way communication that otherwise may never occur. In addition, middle-aged people may feel they reside on an isolated island of responsibility for their parents and for their children. The drain of the expenses, time and emotional fatigue is viewed as a burden.

TIPS FOR SUCCESSFUL UTILIZATION OF REMINISCENCE

1. The past may help deal with the reality of the present.
2. Romance may provide foundation for detailed memories.

3. Reminiscence may provide meaning for those who have little or no future — the very old, ill and infirm.

4. The therapeutic orientation may use past experiences to regenerate or perhaps recreate interests from the past — or even new interests; i.e., interest in plants (Horticulture therapy), music (Music Therapy), historical events, and the use of old films such as Boggie and Bacall.

5. Discussion of past social and professional functions, interests and pleasures may be utilized to create present family understanding and rapport. The Army sergeant and plant managers were groomed to give orders. Everyone listened, obeyed and did not question. Therefore, this may help the family understand that the same traits which generated family economic success also generated the rogue that views himself to be in the captain's chair.

6. Areas which may become a family focus: Holidays, vacations, family pets, animals, perverted interest of certain family members, sports, achievement of certain members, past crises, successes, clothing, autos, boats, dating, or even musical instruments.

7. Emphasis on family self-help, must include the value and limitations of group reminiscence and its dependence upon family communication. All members of the family have impact and value. If one believes, "Even the dog is more valued than I am," the family must decide what can be done about this problem. This is a problem effecting the family system and should be treated as "everyone's" problem.

8. A video tape, journal, or notes of each discussion can be used as a starting point for the next session of therapy.

9. Reminiscence may assist with the natural mourning process and may provide the introspection needed to move towards a new future.

10. Reminiscence can be used to stimulate cognition and clear thinking.

Reminiscence strategies may be used to supplement existing systemic intervention techniques. For some therapists, this may offer alternatives previously unexplored. Just as a life review may add to individual historical insight so may a family reflect upon the past as a positive, productive, therapeutic experience.

REFERENCES

Butler, R. (1963). The life review: An interpretation of reminiscence in the aged. Psychiatry, 26(1) 65-76.

Fallots, R.D. (1980). The impact on mood of verbal reminiscing in later adulthood. International Journal of Aging and Human Development, 10(4) 385-400.

Havighurst, R.J. and Glasser, R. (1972). An exploratory study of reminiscence. Journal of Gerontology, 27(2) 245-253.

Hughston, G.A. and Merrian, S.B. (1982). Reminiscence: a nonformal technique for improving cognitive functioning in the aged. International Journal of Aging and Human Development, 15(2) 139-149.

Keller, J.F. and Hughston, G.A. (1981). Counseling the elderly: a systems approach. Harper and Row.

Lewis, C.N. (1971). Reminiscing and self-concept in old age. Journal of Gerontology, 26(2) 240-243.

Lieberman, M.A. and Falk, J.M. (1971). The remembered past as a source of data for research on the life cycle. Human Development. 14 132-141.

McMahon, A.W. and Rhudick, P.J. (1964). Reminiscing: Adaptational significance in the aged. Archives of General Psychiatry, 10(3) 292-298 (March).

PAVL. (54-58 A.D.) Revised Standard Edition, Oxford annotated Bible, 1965, NY Oxford University Press. 1359-1360.

Snyder, M. and White, P. (1982). Mood and memories: Elation, depression and the remembering of the events of one's life. Journal of Personality, 50(2) 149-167.

Toffler, A. (1970). Future Shock. A Bantam Book.

A Life Systems Approach
to Understanding
Parent-Child Relationships
in Aging Families

Roberta Greene

SUMMARY. This article explores the stresses and strains that may occur between the elderly members of the family and their adult children, particularly those associated with caregiving. It also examines clinical treatment methods from a family systems perspective. Family therapy with older adults and their families is presented as a method which involves the family in problem resolution and emphasizes the therapist role in mobilizing the family system on behalf of the older adult; promoting positive interdependence is seen as a major goal of therapy.

INTRODUCTION

This article explores the stresses and strains that may occur between the elderly members of the family and their adult children, particularly those associated with caregiving. It also examines clinical treatment methods from a family systems perspective.

Despite the widespread acceptance of family therapy as a beneficial mode of treatment, intergenerational forms of family therapy are relatively in their infancy. Throughout the 1960s and 1970s the family treatment unit was generally defined in terms of the nuclear family, namely the recognized relationship between husband and wife and their minor children. The grandparental generation was in

Roberta Greene, PhD, MSW, is Associate Professor and Department Chair, University of Maryland, Department of Social Work, 5401 Wilkens Avenue, Baltimore, MD 21228.

large measure ignored. Pessimistic views of the later stages of life prevailed with most older persons being pictured as isolated or rejected by their families (Butler, 1982; Greene, 1986; Walsh, 1980).

These practice trends were countered by a burgeoning of research information related to family functioning, filial relationships, and the biopsychosocial processes of aging. This provided overwhelming evidence of the reciprocal interaction among generations across the family's life cycle. Personality theorists also addressed the intergenerational nature of family functioning. They spoke to the connecting link between generations based on loyalty, reciprocity and indebtedness. During the 1980s this growing interest has culminated in the recognition of the need to address such family dynamics through the development of intergenerational family therapy models (Eyde & Rich, 1983; Greene, 1986; Silverstone & Burack-Weiss, 1983).

The 1980s have seen an increasing recognition that family treatment approaches are important in ameliorating the problems associated with aging, and more and more practitioners joining the ranks of dedicated mental health professionals working with the aged and their families. However, dramatic changes in the age and social structure of the U. S. population have made it even more critical to further close the gap between what is known about family functioning and clinical practice.

First, life expectancy has increased dramatically over the last decades. Second, the number of older people has increased rapidly and continues to do so. By the year 2025, a projected 19 percent of the total U.S. population will be over 65 years of age. An increasing proportion will be 75 plus. Third, family size has become smaller and smaller. Fourth, three and four generation families are increasingly the norm. Increased longevity and a growing number of three and four generation families means that four-fifths of all people over the age of 65 have children, about half have great-grandchildren, and 10% have a child who is also elderly (NRTA-AARP, 1981).

These demographic forces make it all but impossible for mental health professionals to ignore the later stages of life and argue for a critical role for family therapists in dealing with parent-child relationships in aging families. Furthering a family treatment orientation to remediating the problems associated with the later life stages remains one of the major mental health challenges of the next decades.

THEORETICAL BACKGROUND

Intergenerational models of family therapy focus on involving the family in problem resolution and stress the therapist role in mobilizing the family system on behalf of the older adult. In large measure, the models are eclectic in nature and treatment techniques have grown out of practice experience. Eyde and Rich (1983), for example, in their model, Psychological Distress in Aging, see the family as an important source of information, "silent, unknowing biographers, indirectly recording life events . . ."(p.45). They propose that families provide the context of psychological distress and offer a sense of continuity about the habits and adaptations of older members. They also suggest that families can assist the therapist in "discerning the complex and subtle changes associated with normal or pathological aging" (p.45).

Greene's (1986) Functional Age Model of Intergenerational Family Treatment addresses the family as a system characterized by a relatively high degree of interdependence. She suggests that the stability of the family as a group can be threatened by changes in the older adult's functional capacities; namely, that when there is a significant change in the older adult's psychological, biological and/or social functioning, one should expect to see some degree of disruption throughout the family system. The aim of therapy is to help family members come to terms with their own feelings about the nature of change and to plan for the current level of functioning of the older relative:

The family group seeking help is usually bewildered by the often sudden turn of events in their lives due to the physical, psychological, and/or social changes that have occurred. They are often confused and frustrated with their own inability to understand, accept, and deal with the problem. The role of the therapist is one of helping to resolve the crisis within the context of the family's developmental history and role expectations. (p.18)

The Auxiliary Function Model of Silverstone and Burack-Weiss (1982, 1983) also examines the problems of the frail elderly within a broad psychological and ecological context. They point out that the "key problem facing the frail, impaired person is not of disease or old age but the effects these conditions have on mental and physical functioning . . ." (p.9). Therapy from this perspective is designed to "counteract the effects of depletion and loss" within a supportive relationship. The major goal is to deal with feelings of helplessness in the face of multiple losses and to convey a sense of hope to the older person and their family.

The models described are among the few that were specifically conceived and intended for therapy with older adults and their families. Therefore they have much to offer the practitioner in the way of specialized knowledge and information about the family of later years. Another important source of methods and techniques is family systems theory. Freeman (1981) suggests that family systems theory provides the theoretical underpinning for understanding *all* family behavior. As such, it is "not limited to certain people" and offers a "different set of strategies for practice" (p.3).

While there are a number of different schools of family therapy, there appears to be a number of common principles which guide practice strategies. The following will serve as a framework for examining the stresses and strains associated with the family of later years and for exploring ways in which these may be addressed in treatment:

1. The family system is adaptive, becoming more complex and organized over time.
2. Family therapy is indicated when the family's ability to perform its basic functions becomes inadequate.
3. Therapy is designed to modify those elements of the family relationship system that are interfering with the life tasks of the family and its members.
4. Family treatment focuses on the impact of one family member's behavior on another.

5. The objective of family therapy is to alleviate the difficulty/ problem through modifying the family structure and patterns of communication and by mobilizing the family as a resource.

FAMILY THERAPY WITH OLDER ADULTS AND THEIR FAMILIES

The Initial Phase

As with all family treatment, the first contacts in intergenerational therapy are critical in establishing the boundaries of treatment. Reaching out to the family, identifying and reframing the problem in family terms, and setting appropriate goals are key tasks. Because many families are not knowledgeable about seeking therapy related to "problems associated with older members," it is even more critical that the therapist quickly set the tone of the helping relationship. Familiarizing the clients with the process of therapy during the initial interview, whether in person or by phone, may often involve straightforward explanations about the need for family participation. "Even though you have expressed concern about your father's situation, I think it is very important for all of us to meet together in order to get the full picture." "I would like to meet with both you and your mother in order to best understand your situation."

Family members seeking help usually express a sense of urgency. More often than not, they do not identify the problem as a family one (Freeman, 1981; Greene, 1986). Therefore, the orientation to the therapy process often becomes the key to how/whether the family continues to work on the problem as a unit.

Families in the later phases of the life cycle, as with other life stages, experience a variety of human problems for which they may seek out a mental health professional. However, there is considerable research evidence to suggest that families usually seek help around a change in the biopsychosocial status/needs of older family members. The precipitating event may include a stroke, the death of a spouse, a broken hip, incontinence, or a dementing illness (Brody, 1985; Greene, 1984).

It is important to remember that families remain the primary source of care for older adults. Cross-sectional data indicates that there are well over 5 million people involved in parent-care at any given time. Family help for older adults encompasses 80% to 90% of the household tasks, transportation and shopping.

Research findings on the effects of adult children engaged in elder care support the view that parent care has become a normative but stressful experience for individuals and families and that it is often associated with financial hardship, declines in physical health, and emotional strain:

> . . . study after study has identified the most pervasive and most severe consequences as being in the realm of emotional strains. A long litany of mental health symptoms such as depression, anxiety, frustration, helplessness, sleeplessness, lowered morale, and emotional exhaustion, are related to restrictions on time and freedom, isolation, conflict from competing demands of various responsibilities, difficulties in setting priorities, and interference with life style and social and recreational activities. (Brody, 1985, p.22)

As can be seen in the following case illustration, the stresses and strains of caregiving make a strong case for family-focused treatment/interventions:

> Background Information: Aunt M. is a 94-year-old widowed Black woman. Following the death of her husband, she came to live with her 92-year-old, bedridden sister, Mrs. S. While Aunt M. has worked outside the home, she has remained with her sister for the last 30 years, providing companionship, support and assistance to all the family. She is identified as the historical family "caregiver."
>
> The S. family was referred (with permission) to a Geriatric Assessment Program by a nephew from out of town. During his visit, he became concerned about the lack of consistent, dependable help with Mrs. S.'s care and the amount of caregiving responsibilities assumed by Aunt M.
>
> Aunt M.'s physical health was reported to be good; while Mrs. S. has been immobile and incontinent for the past two years. She requires assistance with all activities of daily liv-

ing. She is, however, mentally alert, and according to her nephew "happy with her living arrangements."

Mrs. S. has three sons who are all college graduates with responsible professional positions. Two live in the area and assist with financial matters, grocery shopping and decision making. The family has also attempted to hire outside help, however, Aunt M. is described as somewhat "intolerable" of strangers in the home, and "exacting" with regard to how she wants things done. As yet, the family has not been able to come together to arrive at a plan. They now question if Aunt M. will be able to continue to provide care for Mrs. S. who now requires constant care and supervision.[1]

Problems associated with parent-care, as seen in the S. family, clearly are complex and multifaceted involving affective and instrumental components. Instrumental problems such as physical health, finances, and/or housekeeping, because they are associated with tasks of daily living, become paramount in the minds of family members. It is not unusual that adult children will first ask for a specific service for the older adult. They also may anticipate that the practitioner will make particular arrangements and/or provide a concrete service such as a home health aid or meals-on-wheels (Greene, 1986). The family first needs to be assured that they will be assisted in obtaining services that they determine with the therapist are necessary. Questions can then be focused on that which requires family organization and planning: Who are the central persons in the family system? How do they perceive the problem? How does the family interact as a group? (Stamm, 1972).

Creating a distinction between requests for concrete versus therapeutic services establishes a false dichotomy. Silverstone and Burack-Weiss (1982) point out that the affective elements of the therapy can actually be the prelude to the instrumental ones; Greene (1986) suggests that the therapist look beyond concrete requests in order to understand how a particular service is perceived by the client family as well as what needs it fulfills. In the case of the S. family, members tended to remain focused on specific service

1. Barbara Soniat, George Washington University, Washington, DC.

needs. Aunt M. found it difficult to express her personal needs and talk about the many burdens of caregiving she was experiencing. Those therapeutic interventions that are coupled with appropriate health and/or social service are most likely to alleviate her stress.

Family systems therapists recognize that the family seeking treatment is experiencing a crisis that challenges its adaptive capacity. This means that the patterns of emotional and social support that the family has developed over the years are tested. It also means that unresolved conflicts surface at this time and enter into the therapeutic situation. Diagnostic clues to such family patterns of interaction can be picked up early in the therapy. In the S. family, the fact that Aunt M. was the primary family caregiver was obtained in the first interview.

A primary issue with which therapists working with the aged and their families must deal centers around the theme of dependence-independence. Most gerontologists agree that helping the family of later years come to terms with the role changes necessary to establish/negotiate a mutually responsible adult parent-child relationship is the bedrock of therapeutic work (Blenkner, 1965; Brody, 1985; Butler & Lewis, 1973; Spark & Brody, 1970). Resolution of such dependency issues in later life, says Walsh (1980, p.206):

> . . . requires a realistic acceptance of strengths and limitations of the older adult, and the ability to allow oneself to be dependent when appropriate. It also requires the adult child's ability to accept a filial role, taking responsibility for what he or she can appropriately do for aging parents, as well as recognition of what he or she cannot do.

As is illustrated by the S. Family, this often stretches the family's ability to integrate loss, to grieve, and to reinvest in the future (Solomon, 1973).

Intergenerational therapy is no different from other forms of family treatment in the respect that problems are first defined as "belonging" to one individual, in this case the older family member. Therefore, reframing the problem in family terms is a critical component of the initial phase of treatment. As the S. family clearly points out this may be difficult. Most families are quick to point out what they perceive as a decline in functioning in the older adult. Questions related to how family roles have been changing over time are particularly useful in trying to achieve a family treatment perspective.

The S. family valued stability, and self-sufficiency.

> Aunt M. had difficulty accepting help from non-family members, and expressed a lot of ambivalence about long term care options. None of the available options — more help in the home, seeking a live-in helper, placing her sister in a nursing home, and possibly relocating to a smaller residence — seemed congruent with her traditional role as family caregiver. Mrs. S.'s sons were accustomed to demanding schedules, and to taking responsibility for decision making. At the same time they expressed guilt that the pressures of their employment commitments did not allow them to assume more responsibility for their mother's care. Whenever a reference was made to Aunt M. being overburdened by caregiving, Victor took on the role of family spokesperson and gatekeeper. At the same time, family members were struggling with feelings of loss because their mother no longer seemed the powerful person she once was.

Helping the family understand how "mother's problem" can have a ripple effect throughout the family system became an initial goal of therapy. Freeman (1981, p.169-170) suggests that it is important for the therapist to pay attention to the following dynamics in order to know best how to reframe the presenting problem:

1. Which family member originally defined the problem?
2. How do members relate to each other and how does the family as a group react to the therapist?
3. Which family member tries hardest to control the problem?
4. Who offers explanations about how the family operates as a social system?

In brief, reframing the problem means that the therapist organizes the assessment/diagnostic information and interprets it in such a way as to facilitate the formulation of a family-focused treatment plan.

Setting goals or formulating a treatment plan with the family, means that there is a mutual agreement about the direction of therapy and follow-up services. For example, the S. family had a relatively fixed idea of how they would use the Geriatric Assessment Program. Any contract made with the family had to take that into account.

Families that come for help "for an older adult" remain in therapy relatively short periods of time. This would indicate that the therapist clearly and quickly establish goals which are aimed at "minimizing the negative effects of the older person's impairment, and increasing the skills and confidence of family members" (Eyde & Rich, 1983).

Implementing Treatment Goals

During the middle phase of therapy, the goal is to mobilize the family system on behalf of its members. The family's treatment potential depends upon its unique constellation and is related to the system it has created over the years. A key question for the therapist working with the S. family is how to address the established roles and at the same time respect the family hierarchy.

Central elements in the family's ability to change/cope (namely, to adjust to new demands and losses) are the unresolved loyalty conflicts and unsettled accounts between first and second-generation family members. Family systems theorists refer to this loyalty or connecting tie between the generations as "reciprocal indebtedness" (Boszormenyi-Nagy & Spark, 1973). Reciprocal indebtedness may take the form of physical caretaking, telephoning, visiting, writing, showing interest, respect and concern.

Brody (1985) postulates that feelings of indebtedness can be a most powerful force in the family of later years and a major source of stress and guilt for adult children. Her studies on women providing parent-care document that a majority of women "somehow" feel guilty that they are not doing enough for their mothers. "The truth," says Brody (p.26) is that adult children cannot and do not provide the same total care to their elderly parents that those parents gave to them in the good old days of their infancy and childhood. The roles of parent and child cannot be reversed in that sense. The good old days, then, may be . . . an earlier period in the individual's and family's history to which there can be no return.

The S. family appears to be tied to the myth and to act out the belief that "somehow" Aunt M. can "do more." Roles become muddied; no one knows who is parent and who is child. This makes it more difficult for the therapist to further adult-to-adult relationships and to mobilize the family system on behalf of Mrs. S.

The essence of the psychological relationship in treatment remains child to parent. In order for the stress on the family to be reduced, interventions during the middle phase of therapy should address this feature of the dependency-independence issue. Spark and Brody (1970, p.6) best express this when they state that "the behavior of a brain-damaged regressed old person may appear child-like but he is not a child. Half a century of adulthood cannot be wiped out."

Bowen's (1972) family systems concept of differentiation of self, which is concerned with the degree of unresolved emotional attachments to one's family of origin, is another that is useful here. He suggests intergenerational therapy take into account that each member of a family exhibits a certain degree of connectedness or differentiation from his/her family of origin. The amount of emotional contact is viewed on a continuum, ranging from those who are emotionally "cut off" to those who are strongly (symbiotically) attached. The degree to which there is viable emotional contact with past generations of the family strongly influences current relationships and obligation. To the extent the therapist can uphold the individuation of each family member and at the same time promote interdependence, the family will become more functional. It could be said that Aunt M. is the adult child who is "most attached" to her family of origin. Perhaps that is why she appears "more committed" to the caregiving role, and her nephews are willing to "surrender" it to her.

Termination

In most forms of treatment, if the early and middle stages of therapy are successful, termination will occur naturally. In intergenerational therapy, a major indicator of success is a more positive interdependence among family members. Adult children are more accepting of what they can and cannot do in the filial role, and all family members have modified their roles accordingly. In situations involving older adults who are frail and/or demented, such as the S. family, the reality is that the family will have to manage needed community resources and continue in the caregiving role. It is important for the therapist to educate and prepare the family to case management services to identify and coordinate a more effective home care plan.

The readiness/ability of families to carry on should be explored during termination. In many agencies this may mean that cases "remain open" after the "therapy or counseling stage" because they need indefinite service. For this reason, feedback to the family and an evaluation of the therapy process are critical elements of the final stage of treatment.

REFERENCES

Blenker, M. (1965). Social work and family relationships in later life with some thoughts on filial maturity. In E. Shanas & G. Streib (Eds.), *Social structure and the family*. Englewood Cliffs, NJ: Prentice-Hall.

Boszormenyi-Nagy, I., & Spark, G. (1973). *Invisible loyalties*. New York: Harper and Row.

Bowen, M. (1966). The use of family theory in clinical practice. *Comprehensive Psychiatry, 7*, 345-374.

Brody, E. (1981). Women in the middle and family help to older people. *The Gerontologist, 21*, 471-480.

Brody, E. (1985). Parent care as a normative family stress. *The Gerontologist, 25(1)*, 19-29.

Butler, R. N., & Lewis, M. (1973). *Aging and Mental Health*. St. Louis, MO: C. V. Mosby Co.

Eyde, D. R., & Rich, J. (1983). *Psychological distress in aging: A family management model*. Rockville, MD: Aspen Publications.

Freeman, D. S. (1981). *Techniques of family therapy*. New York: Jason Aronson.

Greene, R. R. (1982). Families and the nursing home social worker. *Social Work in Health Care, 7(3)*, 57-67.

Greene, R. R., Lebow, G., & Daylyn, H. (1984). The use of long-term care resources in an ethnic community. *The Gerontologist, 24*, 307.

Greene, R. R. (1986). *Social work with the aged and their families*. Hawthorene, NY: Aldine De Gruyter.

NRTA-AARP (National Retired Teachers Association-American Association of Retired Persons) (1981). National survey of older Americans.

Silverstone, B., & Burack-Weiss, A. (1982). The social work function in nursing homes and home care. *Journal of Gerontological Social Work, 5(1/2)*, 7-33.

Silverstone, B., & Burack-Weiss, A. (1983). *Social work practice with the frail elderly and their families*. Springfield, IL: Charles C Thomas.

Solomon, M. (1973). A developmental conceptual premise for family therapy. *Family Process, 12*, 179-188.

Spark, G. (1974). Grandparents and intergenerational family therapy. *Family Process, 13*, 225-237.

Spark, G., & Brody, E. (1972). The aged are family members. In C. Sager & H. Kaplan (Eds.), *Progress in group and family therapy*, (pp. 712-725). New York: Brunner Mazel Publishers.

Stamm, I. (1972). Family therapy. In F. Hallis, (Ed.), *Casework: A psycho-social therapy*. New York: Random House.

Walsh, F. (1980). The family in later life. In E. A. Carter & M. McGoldrick, (Eds.), *The family life cycle: A framework for family therapy*. New York: Gardner Press, Inc.

Family Caregiving and Aging: Strategies for Support

Vicki L. Schmall
Clara C. Pratt

SUMMARY. Increasingly families face difficult dilemmas and decisions when elderly relatives become dependent and need the assistance of others. This article discusses the demographic and social trends which impact on the ability of families to provide the needed support and the stresses individuals can experience when providing care. Four strategies that can enhance a family's effectiveness to make decisions and their ability to provide caregiving are discussed. These are educational programs, family conferences, support groups, and respite care.

A 65-year-old son says, "Dad is so unsteady on his feet. He shouldn't live alone. He's fallen twice this past week. I'm scared that the next time he falls he'll seriously hurt himself and not be found for hours or days. He refuses help and won't consider moving."

Grace, 77, is emotionally and physically exhausted from providing care to her husband, 80, who has Alzheimer's disease. During the last three years she has left their home only to get necessities.

Vicki L. Schmall, PhD, is Associate Professor, and Extension Gerontology Specialist, Oregon State University Extension Service, 161 Miiam Hall, Corvallis, OR 97331-5106. Correspondence should be directed to her. Clara C. Pratt, PhD, is Associate Professor, Human Development and Family Studies, College of Home Economics, Oregon State University, Corvallis, OR 97331-5106.

Martha, 48, feels overwhelming guilt for placing her mother in a nursing home. She says, "my family has always taken care of our own. I'm the first to fail in my duty."

What should I do with Dad? Should Mom be allowed to remain in her own home even though I feel it is no longer safe? How can I get Dad to accept help? How do I balance my responsibilities to my parent, spouse, children, job . . . and what about me? These are just a few of the difficult situations and questions families increasingly face. Although the majority of older adults live independently, with advancing age and declining health, limited resources, or death of a spouse, many need some assistance from family.

CHANGING DEMOGRAPHICS

Changing population trends are placing unprecedented strain on the ability of families to support and care for their older family members (Polisar and Bengston, 1984). Not only are more people reaching age 65 than ever before, the very old (age 85 and older), are the fastest growing age group in the United States (U.S. Senate, 1984).

The growth of the oldest of the old is particularly significant because this is the group of elderly who are most likely to experience dependency on others. According to national surveys, nearly 23 percent of the elderly are functionally disabled, requiring assistance with personal care, mobility, activities of daily living, or nursing care (Doty, 1986). Although fewer than one in 10 persons age 65-74 requires help, four in 10 who are 85 or older need assistance (Feller, 1983). Eighty percent of these dependent elderly are able to live in the community, as opposed to a nursing home, because of the support received from family and friends.

Providing long-term care to frail, dependent elders is increasingly a common experience for individuals and families (Brody, 1985). Although the myth of "family abandonment" would have us believe that families do not take care of their older family members as well as they did "in the good old days," the reality is that families today provide more care, more difficult care, and care over a longer period of time to more family members than has ever been the case before (Brody, 1985). For some women, as many years will be spent caring for a dependent parent or spouse as was spent caring for a dependent child.

The ability of a family to provide needed care can be complicated by several factors, including mobility, declining birth rate, employment of women, and divorce and remarriage. Geographic distance can make it more difficult for a family to provide continuing assistance to a frail, impaired elder. Some families find themselves driving or flying back and forth to repeated crises or spending long weekends or vacations "getting things in order" or "checking on Mom or Dad." Such long distance managing takes not only time and money, but can be emotionally and physically exhausting as well. Because of lower birth rates, there are also more older people with fewer family members to provide support and assist with decision-making (Polisar and Bengston, 1984).

Studies by Cicerelli (1983) suggest that divorce, separation and widowhood among adult children is associated with elderly parents receiving fewer types of care. Furthermore, more adults today have living parents, grandparents and great-grandparents than ever before.

Women have been the traditional caregivers. However, the trend toward women entering the labor force complicates their capacity to meet the needs of frail older family members (Doty, 1986). Research findings, however, on the impact of female employment on family caregiving have been contradictory. Many employed women provide as much support to aged relatives as their nonemployed counterparts. What they tend to give up is time for themselves.

Increasingly it's not only middle-aged adults who are concerned about supporting aged parents, but also the "old adult children" — people in their sixties, seventies, and even eighties. Currently, 10 percent of the population age 65 and older have children who are also 65 years of age or older (Brody, 1985). Because of longer lifespans and survival of persons with previously life-ending diseases, more and more individuals are providing care simultaneously to two or more disabled elders.

TYPES OF CAREGIVING

Caregiving can evolve over a long period of time, or occur suddenly as in the case of a stroke or accident. A family may adjust better to caregiving demands when the relative's need for assistance increases gradually versus when a sudden need results from an acute health crisis which produces a sudden drop in the person's functional ability (Harkins, 1985). Although short-term caregiving can be stressful, stress tends to be highest when caregiving is prolonged over months or years, the ill person's needs are increasing, and the caregiver feels he or she receives little or no support.

Caring for a person who has a dementing illness such as Alzheimer's disease can be particularly stressful. The person not only requires increasing assistance and supervision as the illness progresses, but also becomes increasingly impaired in language, reasoning ability, memory and social behavior (Gwyther, 1987). One of the most difficult aspects of coping with a progressive, dementing illness is losing the person you've always known, even though the person is physically alive. As one woman said, "I've already watched the death of my husband. Now I'm watching the death of the disease."

Contrary to popular belief, nursing home placement does not necessarily relieve a caregiver's feeling of stress. Studies show that feelings of burden experienced by caregivers to institutionalized elders are nearly identical to those of community-dwelling elderly, although the sources of the burden shift (Pratt, Schmall and Wright, 1987a). Many injunctions continue to exist against placement, and as a result, a caregiver may feel a sense of failure, even when placement is the best choice. Stress may also result from difficult visits, traveling to and from the care facility, family conflicts regarding placement, and the cost of financing care.

IMPACT OF CAREGIVING

Caregiving involves many changes for the caregiver as well as the care receiver. The direction, amount and nature of aid patterns between parent and child generally changes from being mutual or reciprocal to a one-way aid pattern. This can be difficult for both the giver and receiver and can cause fear, anger, conflict and confusion

(Archbold, 1980). The care receiver may become depressed because of his or her inability to contribute to the family as before and fear becoming a burden. The caregiver, on the other hand, may experience role overload, constriction of former activities, increased isolation and reduced financial resources.

Parental disability can also threaten the relationship that had previously been established between parent and child. Where caregiving involves increased contact, such contact can be particularly difficult where a relationship survived because of "distancing" that had been created. Tobin and Kulys (1979) also found that aged parents were more likely to label themselves as being "closest to" their child before caregiving, but not afterwards.

Caregivers frequently find themselves pulled by the many roles they play—parent, spouse, employee, and adult child. There simply may not be enough time and energy to meet all demands. The potential for role conflict is particularly great for middle-aged women who provide child and elder care simultaneously. Marital and family problems can arise if time spent providing care to elderly relatives means a couple's and family's time together and social and recreational activities are severely curtailed. Caregivers frequently report struggling with the ethical question of "to whom do I owe" the most time, energy and attention (Pratt, Schmall and Wright, 1987b).

In addition, many women "in the middle" are also employed. A national study (National Survey, 1982) found one out of ten caregivers leave the labor force to assume care for an older relative. Among those who continue to work, many rearrange work schedules, reduce work hours, or take time off without pay.

Caregivers frequently become increasingly isolated. Restriction of one's personal activities and social life is one of the most frequently cited problems among caregivers to moderately and severely impaired elders (Zarit, 1987). Becoming isolated in one's home can result in a person feeling "trapped" or a "prisoner of love." Maintaining contact with friends and involvement in outside activities is critical for a caregiver's well-being.

Caregivers frequently struggle to balance their expectations for themselves with what they can actually achieve. Sometimes caregivers expect too much of themselves and get into a state of constant anxiety or worry because they think they are not doing what they should. Female caregivers are particularly vulnerable to the "shoulds" and often believe they should be able to do everything themselves (Pratt et al., 1987b). When unable to do so, they often feel guilty or depressed (Schmall and Stiehl, 1987).

Readjusting one's expectations of an ill family member also can be difficult, particularly when the person was a strong, independent person, exercised control, or was the family decision-maker. Readjusting such expectations is particularly difficult if the caregiver's own identity is strongly tied to who their family member was. However, hanging on to who the person was and what the person could do but now no longer can, leaves a caregiver open to a continual, prolonged grieving.

One of the greatest stresses of caregiving can be the emotional strain. In addition to observing a loved one deteriorate in function, many other factors can contribute to emotional strain. These include disagreements among family members about care arrangements, lack of needed support from family and friends, a poor relationship between the ill person and caregiver prior to caregiving, and the ill relative's personality and expectations (Zarit, 1987; Schmall and Stiehl, 1987). Some older people have been difficult all of their lives and may be even more so when they need the support of others. As one woman said, "The hardest thing for me is not being able to please Mom. No matter what I do, she criticizes how I do it or makes me feel I never do enough." Almost every caregiver experiences a wide range of emotions, some of which are powerful, uncomfortable, conflicting and confusing.

For some caregivers, financial concerns are a major source of stress. One spouse said, "The greatest worry I have is I have used up the last of the money we received from the sale of the house. Now we will be using up our small store of stocks and bonds . . . then, who will look after me." A daughter stated, "I interrupted my career for eight years to care for my mother. Not only did I lose a salary during that time . . . my retirement income is considerably smaller than it would have been had I continued working." Competent financial and legal advice can make the difference between economic survival and destitution (Gilfix, 1984; Pratt, Nay, Ladd and Heagerty, in press).

A caregiver's perception of his or her caregiving situation may be more important in determining the degree of stress than the amount of actual change or disruption. For example, Archbold (1980) found that families who did not perceive their relative's stroke as disruptive reported less stress than families who did.

STRATEGIES TO ENHANCE FAMILY DECISION-MAKING AND CAREGIVING

A woman writing in a local newspaper stated, "Those of us who are responsible for our aging parents, making decisions about how they should be cared for, somehow just muddle through. And, as a result, I think many of us make some serious mistakes." A major role for the practitioner is to provide families with the information and skills that will help reduce some of those "serious mistakes."

Agencies are generally more likely to provide services such as in-home assistance and meals-on-wheels to persons living alone than to persons living with a family member (Archbold, 1980). The assumption is frequently made that the "relatives can do it." However, families have limited resources. If agencies are going to fully meet the needs of elderly clients, the family also must be viewed as client. Conducting an assessment of the caregiver's situation and needs can be just as important as the assessment of the older person's needs. A family's willingness to provide care is not always indicative of ability to do so.

Four strategies that can enhance a family's effectiveness to make decisions and their ability to provide caregiving will be discussed: educational programs, family conferences, support groups, and respite care.

Education

All too often, families find themselves faced with wondering, "What would Mom (or Dad) have wanted?" Accurate information, advance planning and decision-making with aging relatives prior to crisis generally result in the best decisions for everyone. A priority recommendation from a conference on aging issues sponsored by the Hogg Foundation for Mental Health was the need to "develop community education programs to assist people in knowing their options about and planning for such issues as their aging process and their financial, health, and housing needs *before* actual decisions have to be made'' (Coleman et al., 1985, p. 27).

Many current education programs rely primarily on the didactic presentation of information, i.e., lecture, frequently followed by an opportunity to ask questions. The best learning situations, however, encourage empathy of the older person and other family members, increase a person's confidence in problem solving, provide help in defining difficult situations, and provide skills for how to marshal social support (Pratt et al., 1985). Since the ability to problem solve and reframe problems often requires experience, programs need to provide an opportunity for participants to practice skills in a non-threatening way.

Interactive and experiential methods can enhance affective learning (Menks, 1983). Simulations are a particularly effective method for helping individuals to better understand age-related changes. By "stepping into the shoes" of an older person, family members gain a greater appreciation of the impact hearing impairment, visual changes, loss of taste and smell sensitivity, limited mobility, and other changes can have on an older person's ability to function, social interactions, and self-esteem. Guides for conducting simulations include *Simulations: A Method for Understanding Physical Changes in Later Life* (Schmall, 1985) and *Sensitizing People to the Processes of Aging: The Inservice Educator's Guide* (Ernst and Shore, 1978).

Many fields of study have developed games to facilitate learning, teach principles or skills, or clarify values (Engs et al., 1975). Recently, gerontology-based educational games also have been developed, including *Families and Aging: Dilemmas and Decisions* (Schmall et al., 1984). During the game, players confront real-life problems, dilemmas, and decisions families face in later life. They are challenged to examine their values and attitudes, to identify alternative approaches to problems, to view issues from the perspective of various family members, and to consider the impact of decisions on everyone. This is done by players being in a variety of roles during game play.

In a group, family members can be hesitant to discuss their situation for fear of "what will others think." It can be less threatening to begin by discussing another family's situation. Media that present an individual's or family's story can help create a less threatening environment for discussion and provide a common frame of reference for problem solving. Examples of such media are *My Mother, My Father, Where Do We Go From Here?* and the four-part slide-tape in the series on caregiving entitled *When Dependency Increases* (Schmall and Stiehl, 1987). Unlike most media, each slide-tape program in the *When Dependency Increases* series includes a comprehensive instructor's guide, overhead transparency masters to guide discussion, presentation techniques, promotional materials, and handouts. Written materials which can be taken home, digested and shared with others are a vital component to any educational program (Gwyther, 1987).

Several guides for conducting either a single program or a series of educational programs are currently available and can reduce a professional's preparation time. These include *When Dependency Increases* (Schmall and Stiehl, 1987), *Families Caring for Elders* (Ragosa and Jackson, 1987), *Family Seminars for Family Caregiving* (University of Washington, 1984), and *As Parents Grow Older: A Program Replication Manual* (Silverman et al., 1981). In recent years, several nationwide newsletters designed specifically for caregivers have been developed: *Advice for Adults with Aging Parents or a Dependent Spouse*, *Parent Care*, *The Later Years*, and *The Caregiver*. These newsletters can provide on-going education to families.

Family Conferences

Although care for an older person may be provided primarily by one person, all family members should be involved in the planning and continual support. The family conference is one strategy for deciding how to share responsibilities.

A family conference should be held as early as possible after the need for caregiving arises. The conference gives everyone an opportunity to discuss caregiving concerns, identify potential problems and solutions, and negotiate the sharing of caregiving tasks. A conference can also clarify each person's expectations and minimize misunderstandings.

Everyone who is concerned and may be affected by care decisions should be involved in the family conference. This includes the older person for whom plans are being made. If serious illness prevents the person from being involved directly, his or her input should be obtained and the person kept informed.

A family member should not be excluded from a family conference because of distance, personality, family history with the older person, or limited resources. It's just as important to include a difficult, argumentative family member, or one who never visits, as it is to involve those who are supportive. This helps to ensure greater success and support for the plan, and helps prevent later undermining of decisions.

Sometimes a two-step conference can be helpful. The first meeting is held without the older person for the purpose of airing ideas and feelings, identifying concerns, looking at gaps in information, and discussing responsibilities for each family member. It is often useful to have each person identify their one major concern. The purpose should not be to make the decision or to "gang up" on the older person. A second meeting is then held with the older person, who is actively involved in assessing all the options and making decisions. Some of the best decisions may be those that involve the least change. Consider this question: What is the smallest change that can be made that would improve the situation? Being as *specific* as possible about problems and solutions is important (see Herr and Weakland, 1979, for further ideas).

A family conference is not always easy, and in some families it is impossible. It's most difficult for families who have never discussed feelings and family concerns. Where conflicts already exist among family members, decision-making is difficult. When family members come together after years of separation, old conflicts can re-emerge with regard to relationships, family roles, expectations, and even inheritance.

Family members often have different perceptions about the care needs of an older person, the best option, the division of care tasks, and how money should be spent. For example, one brother might not want his parent's resources—his potential inheritance—spent for in-home services or nursing home care. He may prefer the family to provide the needed care, while another brother feels, "Mom's money is there to spend on her" and prefers to purchase services. Because of these differing perceptions an objective third party, skilled in working with the elderly and their families, can help increase the success of a family conference. Some practitioners and agencies are offering "family consultation services" that include facilitation of family meetings (Herr and Weakland, 1979).

Support Groups

Most people benefit from sharing their feelings and situations with someone who is supportive and listens nonjudgmentally. In some areas, mutual support groups have developed for this kind of sharing. Some groups are oriented to specific diseases like cancer, Parkinson's disease, lung disease, or Alzheimer's disease and other dementias. Others are for family caregivers in general.

Support groups can help normalize the experience of caregivers and help them feel "I am not alone" (Rzetelny and Mellor, 1981). They give an opportunity to share openly with others who understand and to learn techniques for coping. For the isolated caregiver deprived of the intimacy and support from their ill family member, it can offer a socially acceptable outlet (Gwyther, 1987). In addition, a support group may be the primary source of advice since some caregivers will not follow a counselor's advice, but will try approaches suggested by another caregiver (Zarit and Zarit, 1982). Levels of burden, however, appear to be more influenced by changes in a person's caregiving situation than by support group participation (George, 1984).

Groups need a skilled facilitator who possesses group process skills as well as knowledge about the issues faced by caregivers. The facilitator can make a major difference in the degree of success of a support group, level of group cohesiveness, and attendance and participation of caregivers.

Some of the most successful groups have co-facilitators — a family caregiver and a community agency professional (Schmall, 1984; Gwyther, 1987). While a single facilitator can be effective, co-facilitators bring a wider range of expertise to a group, can collaborate on planning and provide feedback to each other (Silverman, 1980). Also, if a group member should become upset and leave the room, one facilitator can leave with the family member and the other person can continue to facilitate the group.

A particular strength of a family member as a co-facilitator is the bringing of personal experience and authenticity to group discussion (Silverman, 1980). A caregiver often can raise issues characteristic of the caregiving situation that may be more difficult for a non-caregiver to articulate.

The professional, on the other hand, provides sanctions, legitimacy and credibility to family members' concerns (Gwyther, 1987). The professional frequently is in a better position to monitor discussion and intervene when conflicts erupt or when a group member dominates discussion or offers a quick, unrealistic solution to a difficult or long-standing problem. A professional also can more appropriately direct a group member to therapy or counseling when a member's needs are beyond a group's capability.

Based on statewide experience in developing numerous support groups, Gwyther (1987) indicates it is best when no given agency is perceived as "owning a support group." This increases the potential for continuous referrals from throughout the community. Some evidence suggests that support groups organized according to the caregivers' relationship (i.e., all spouses or all children) tend to be more effective than when spouses and adult children are mixed together (Zarit, 1987).

Some people initially find coming to a session labeled "support group" threatening because they feel their situations and feelings are unique or they are reluctant to disclose their concerns to anyone other than a professional. An educational program or series can be an effective springboard for developing a support group. An essential component of such programs is to plan for a social break. Participants generally make contact and have informal sharing during such breaks, which can help make a support group appear less threatening.

Although support groups are beneficial, they are not effective for everyone. In his research of caregivers to Alzheimer patients, Zarit (1987) found that approximately one-third of caregivers in support groups experienced increased burden as a result of participation. He stated, "Our findings suggest that, on the average, caregivers receiving individual counseling find more benefit in that than in support groups; they get more insight into the problem and feel more support. They value the relationship with the counselor more" (Zarit, 1987, p. 118). Although support groups may work very well for some caregivers, individual counseling may be better for others, particularly for persons experiencing high stress.

Resources for developing and maintaining support groups include: *The Duke Aging Center Family Support Program* (Gwyther, 1987); *Mobilizing Networks of Mutual Support: How to Develop Alzheimer Caregivers' Support Groups* (Gwyther and Brooks, 1983); *Mutual Help Groups: Organization and Development* (Silverman, 1980); *It Doesn't Just Happen: What Makes a Support Group Good?* (Schmall, 1984); *Support Groups for Caregivers of the Aged* (Rzetelny and Mellor, 1981); and *Caregiver Support Groups* (Lidoff and Beaver, 1984).

Respite Services

Studies suggest that families are better able to tolerate long-term caregiving for a disabled elderly person—particularly one afflicted with a dementing illness or who requires heavy personal care—if they are able to obtain respite care, i.e., temporary relief from caregiving responsibilities (Doty, 1986). Although the primary intended beneficiary of respite services is the caregiver, the ill person also benefits (Crozier, 1982). In many cases, a respite care provider may be the only outside-the-family socialization the elder receives.

Respite services may be provided in-home or out-of-home; for a few hours, a day, overnight, weekends, or longer; on a planned or emergency basis; by paid staff or trained volunteers. In-home respite care can include companion-type or supervision services or the temporary use of homemaker and/or home health services. Out-of-home care includes adult day care or short stays in adult foster care homes, nursing homes, or hospitals. In many communities, such formal respite services are limited or not available.

Many caregivers seek respite care much too late—when they are in crisis, desperate, or their family member is severely debilitated and requires care beyond the skill of respite workers. Respite is most beneficial when obtained early in caregiving and used as a preventive measure. The purpose of respite is to prevent caregiver burnout, not treat it. Dunn (1988) suggests that one reason respite may be viewed as a "service of last resort," is that many publicly funded or subsidized respite programs limit access to families caring for an individual "at risk of institutionalization." The message given to caregivers may be: "Respite is a service when you are having trouble coping or the condition of your loved one is progressing to the point where placement may be necessary" (Dunn, p. 2).

Many caregivers are fiercely independent and feel "I should be able to care for my family member myself." or "No one can care for him like I can." As a result, they are reluctant to accept help. It often helps to encourage caregivers to view their need for a break in caregiving as a consequence of difficult circumstances, not as inadequacy on their part. Some caregivers are apprehensive about leaving the person with a "stranger" or having a stranger in their home. Careful orientation of both the patient and caregiver, and educational and service activities that create a feeling of a family-respite team can help alleviate some of these apprehensions.

Women appear to have more difficulty purchasing respite care. Bader (1985) suggests women may be buying into the assumption that "caregiving is women's work." Men, on the other hand, may feel less secure in the caregiving role, feeling they do not have the needed skills to "take care of someone else." Thus, they are more willing to hire help.

Even when formal respite services are not available, professionals play a vital role in encouraging caregivers to take breaks in caregiving and helping them to identify and overcome barriers to obtaining respite. Members of the caregiver's informal support system may be able to provide respite when formal services do not exist or are not accessible. However, some caregivers need help to reach out and ask for assistance, particularly those who view asking for help as a sign of weakness, helplessness, inadequacy or failure. A physician, by writing a "prescription for respite" for so many hours a week or month, can often provide the authority a caregiver may need to begin respite (Dunn, 1988).

Resources for developing respite programs include the Respite Companion Model Program (Lidoff, 1983), *Respite Care for the*

Frail Elderly (Foundation for Long Term Care, 1983), and *How to Manual on Providing Respite Care for Family Caregivers* (Project Share, 1985).

CONCLUSION

In the past, public policy and programs have been directed primarily toward the older person needing assistance and have neglected the needs of the family caregiver. However, if families are to provide care, attention must also be directed to the stresses caregivers experience and their needs. Support must preserve the caregiver's, as well as the care-receiver's, health and well-being.

REFERENCES

Advice for Adults with Aging Parents or a Dependent Spouse, Helping Publications, P.O. Box 339, Glenside, PA 19038.

Archbold, P. 1980. Impact of parent-caring on middle-aged offspring. *Journal of Gerontological Nursing* 6(2):78-84.

Bader, J. 1985. Respite care: Temporary relief for caregivers. *Women and Health* 10(2/3):39-52.

Brody, E. 1985. Parent care as a normative family stress. *The Gerontologist* 25(1):19-29.

Cicerelli, V. 1983. A comparison of helping behavior to elderly parents of adult children with intact and disrupted marriages. *The Gerontologist* 23:619-625.

Coleman, M., Smith, B., and Warren, C. 1985. *Looking Forward: Texas and Its Elderly*. Austin, TX, University of Texas.

Crozier, M. 1982. Respite care keep elders at home longer. *Perspective on Aging* 11(5), September/October.

Doty, P. 1986. Family care of the elderly: the role of public policy. *The Milbank Quarterly* 64(1):34-75.

Dunn, L. 1987. Respite: preventing burnout. *Advice* 2(6):2-4.

Engs, R. C., Barnes, S. E., and Wantz, M. 1975. *Health Games Students Play: Creative Strategies for Health Education*. Dubuque, IA, Kendall/Hunt Publishing Co.

Ernst, M. and Shore, E. 1978. *Sensitizing People to the Processes of Aging: The Inservice Educators Guide*. Denton, TX, Center for Studies on Aging.

Feller, B. 1983. Americans need help to function at home. *Advanced Data*, No. 92, September 14, 1983.

Foundation for Long Term Care. 1983. *Respite Care for the Frail Elderly*. Albany, NY, Center for the Study of Aging.

George, L. K. 1984. The burden of caregiving: how much? what kinds? for whom? *Center Reports on Advances in Research* 8(2).

Gilfix, M. 1984. Legal strategies for patients and families. *Generations* 9(2): 46-68.

Gwyther, L. 1987. The Duke Aging Center Family Support Program: a grassroots outreach program generates principles and guidelines. *Center Reports on Advances in Research* 11(2).

Gwyther, L. and Brooks, B. 1983. Mobilizing Networks of Mutual Support: How to Develop Alzheimer's Caregivers' Support Groups. Durham, NC, Duke University for the Study of Aging and Human Development.

Harkins, E. 1985. Family Support and Costs of Services for the Frail Elderly: Final Report. HCFA grant. Richmond, VA, Virginia Commonwealth University.

Herr, J. and Weakland, J. 1979. *Counseling elders and their families: practical techniques for applied gerontology*. New York, NY, Springer.

Lidoff, L. 1983. *Respite Companion Program Model*. Washington, DC, The National Council on the Aging.

Lidoff, L. and Beaver, L. 1984. *Caregiver Support Groups*. Washington, DC, National Council on the Aging.

Menks, F. 1983. The use of a board game to simulate the experiences of old age. *The Gerontologist* 23(6):565-568.

Montgomery, R. 1984. *Family Seminars for Caregiving: Helping Families Help*. Seattle, WA, University of Washington, Pacific Northwest Long-Term Care Center.

My Mother, My Father. Terra Nova Films, 9848 S. Winchester Avenue, Chicago, IL 60643.

National Survey describes caregivers. 1987. *Parent Care* 2(3):1-2. March/April 1987.

Parent Care, Gerontology Center, 316 Strong Hall, University of Kansas, Lawrence, KS 66045.

Polisar, D. and Bengston, V. L. 1984. Population processes and intergenerational relations. In *Family support and Long Term Care*. Excelsior, MN, Interstudy.

Pratt, C., Nay, T., Ladd, L. and Heagerty, B. (in press). Legal-financial education for family caregivers to neurologically impaired older adults. *The Gerontologist*.

Pratt, C., Schmall, V., Wright, S. and Cleland, M. 1985. Burden and coping strategies of caregivers to Alzheimer's patients. *Family Relations: Journal of Applied Child and Family Studies* 34(1):27-34.

Pratt, C., Schmall, V., and Wright, S. 1987a. Burden, coping and health status: a comparison of family caregivers to community-dwelling and institutionalized dementia patients. *Journal of Gerontological Social Work* 10(1/2):99-112.

Pratt, C., Schmall, V., and Wright, S. 1987b. Ethical concerns of family caregivers to dementia patients. *The Gerontologist* 27(5):632-638.

Project Share. 1985. *How to Manual on Providing Respite Care for Family Caregivers*. Rockville, MD, Project Share.

Ragosa, L. and Jackson, R. 1987. *Families Caring for Elders*. Burlington, VT, University of Vermont Extension Service.

Rzetelny, H. and Mellor, J. 1981. *Support Groups for Caregivers of the Aged*. New York, NY, The Natural Supports Program, Community Service Agency.

Schmall, V. 1984. It doesn't just happen: what makes a support group good? *Generations* 9(2):64-67.

Schmall, V. 1985. *Simulations: A method for Understanding Physical Changes in Later Life*. Corvallis, OR, Oregon State University Extension Service.

Schmall, V., Staton, M., and Weaver, D. 1984. *Families and Aging: Dilemmas and Decisions*. Corvallis, OR, Oregon State University Extension Service.

Schmall, V. and Stiehl, R. 1987. *When Dependency Increases*. Corvallis, OR, Oregon State University Extension Service.

Silverman, A. G., Brahce, C. I., and Zielinski, C. 1981. *As Parents Grow Older: A Manual for Program Replication*. Ann Arbor, University of Michigan, Institute of Gerontology.

Silverman, P. 1980. *Mutual Help Groups: Organization and Development*. Beverly Hills, Sage Publications.

The Caregiver. Family Support Program, Center for the Study of Aging and Human Development, Box 2914, Duke University Medical Center, Durham, NC 27710.

The Later Years. Dunn and Hargitt, Inc., 22 N. 2nd Street, Lafayette, IN 47902.

Tobin, S. and Kulys, R. 1979. The family and services. In *Annual Review of Gerontology and Geriatrics* ed. by C. Eisdorfer, 370-399. New York, NY, Springer.

U. S. Senate Special Committee on Aging. 1984. *Aging America: Trends and Projections*. Washington, DC.

Where Do We Go From Here? Education Development Center, 33 Chapel Street, Newton, MA 02160.

Zarit, S. 1987. The burdens of caregiving. In *Confronting Alzheimer's Disease* ed. by A.C. Kalicki. Washington, DC, American Association of Homes for the Aging.

Zarit, S. and Zarit, J. 1982. Families under stress: interventions for caregivers of senile dementia patients. *Psychotherapy: Theory, Research and Practice* 19(4):461-471.

Reversible Mental Illness:
The Role of the Family
in Therapeutic Context

Gregory L. Schmidt

SUMMARY. Family interactions play a significant role in the detection and outcome of psychiatric illness in the elderly. In the evaluation process, the clinician must diagnose both the patient's problems and the family dynamics with regard to the symptomatic presentation. Development of the therapeutic alliance for the entire family and resolution of potentially destructive psychodynamic interactions among family members are the essential work of treating an older adult with a psychiatric illness. Such a family-oriented approach provides the highest probability of a good outcome of treatment.

In recent years, the involvement of family members in the problems of relatives with Alzheimer's disease has been widely reported. Family support is known to be the critical factor which can prevent the institutionalization of a demented patient (Bergmann et al., 1978). A range of services which provide support, education, and psychotherapy for family caregivers has been developed (Schmidt and Keyes, 1985). However, beyond Alzheimer's disease, there is a whole realm of psychiatric illness in the elderly for which interventions with the family can be effective.

The relative lack of literature which addresses family therapy of elderly patients can be traced to the more fundamental problem of lack of societal awareness of treatable psychiatric illness in late life.

Gregory L. Schmidt, MD, PhD, is Assistant Professor of Psychiatry, University of Wisconsin Medical School, Milwaukee Clinical Campus.

89

The long prevalent view that the changes in mood, thought, or behavior in an older adult were the result of normal effects of aging has dissuaded mental health professionals from dealing with the elderly. Another major factor has been a strong bias against psychotherapy for older adults, produced in large part by cognitive and empathic resistances in psychotherapists (Lewis and Johanson, 1982). It is now becoming clear that the entire range of effective psychiatric interventions, family therapy among them, can be a benefit to the older adult.

The purpose of this paper is the discussion of reversible mental illness in the elderly. It begins with an overview of the common psychiatric problems which affect the elderly, presents information regarding prevalence and etiology of these illnesses, and discusses approaches to treatment. It then focuses on the family's role in recognition and understanding of their relative's psychiatric problems and the ways in which a psychotherapist can assist the family to effect successful therapeutic intervention.

DEMENTIA

Dementia, the loss of cognitive abilities and memory function, is primarily a disease of the elderly. While Alzheimer's disease has received the most attention, it is important to realize that 30 to 50% of apparent dementia results from other diseases (Rabins, 1983; Larson et al., 1984). Of the total, about 20% of all dementia is potentially reversible. In these cases, the cognitive impairment results from depression and other psychiatric illness, subdural hematoma, normal pressure hydrocephalus, drug toxicity, benign mass lesion, or hypothyroidism. Specific treatment exists for all of these conditions. Treatment of depression is discussed in the following section. Subdural hematoma, mass lesions, and some cases of normal pressure hydrocephalus respond to neurosurgical approaches. Thyroid hormone replacement can reverse symptoms of hypothyroidism and changes in medication can reduce symptoms of dementia secondary to drug toxicity. The critical issue here is the recognition that cognitive impairment and memory loss in late life may be treatable and thus cannot be written off as normal effects of aging or as symptoms of Alzheimer's disease.

AFFECTIVE DISORDERS

Symptoms of depression are very common in the elderly. Blazer and Williams (1980) studied a community population age 65 and older and found that the rate of dysphoric symptomatology was 14.7%. Of the total population, 3.7% met diagnostic criteria for a major depressive disorder. Later studies as part of the Epidemiological Catchment Area study of the National Institutes of Mental Health have indicated that the six month prevalence rate of major depressive disorder was about 1% in people over 65 (Weissman et al., 1985). In addition to depressed mood, classic symptoms of a major depressive disorder include decreased sleep, decreased appetite, psychomotor changes, decreased energy, decreased self-esteem, complaints of memory and concentration problems, and thoughts of death.

As many of these symptoms can be the result of illness, a premature diagnosis of major depressive disorder may actually prevent the physician from suspecting an underlying cause. Such causes include thyroid disease, cerebrovascular accidents. Parkinson's disease, congestive heart failure, uremia, and malignant disease. Many drugs such as antihypertensives, digoxin, L-dopa, corticosteroids, and estrogens can also produce depressive symptoms.

The classic symptoms of mania—elevated mood, hyperactivity, rapid speech, flight of ideas, grandiosity, and decreased need for sleep—are very difficult to miss. As with major depressive disorder, onset of these symptoms can be the result of medical conditions, especially cerebrovascular accidents and intracranial masses. In all forms of affective disorder, the family's awareness of their relative's medical treatment is critical to helping the physician diagnose such underlying problems.

Once causative medical conditions have been ruled out, tricyclic antidepressants are effective in treating major depressive disorder, and lithium carbonate and antipsychotic medications in treating mania. For major depressive disorder and less severe depression, psychotherapy adds significant benefit to treatment.

PARANOIA AND SCHIZOPHRENIA

In the Epidemiological Catchment Area study, the six month prevalence of schizophrenia in the elderly was 0.3% (Weissman, 1985). That this rate is lower than the 1% of the total population felt to be affected by schizophrenia probably results from the fact that most schizophrenics over 65 are cared for in institutional settings. Elderly patients with less severe symptoms similar to those of schizophrenia are relatively common. Eisdorfer has described a spectrum of severity from suspiciousness through paranoia to schizophrenia (Eisdorfer, 1980). The syndrome of paranoia or late paraphrenia is known to account for about 10% of psychiatric admissions of people over 65 in England (Blessed and Watson, 1982). In this condition, paranoid delusions are present in the absence of the cognitive impairment of dementia or the deterioration of personality seen as schizophrenia. This condition can be treated effectively with antipsychotic medication.

ANXIETY

Fluctuations in the level of anxiety are a normal part of human experience. However, persistent anxiety not clearly related to specific events requires medical and psychiatric attention. Again, medical causes such as hyperthyroidism, hypoglycemia, and caffeine toxicity from medications and beverages must be considered and treated, if present. However, most anxiety in the elderly, like most depression, results from psychosocial factors. Two of the most common factors encountered in the elderly are fear of physical or mental debilitation, and fear of death of self or of a spouse. While there is a role for antianxiety medication in symptom control, psychotherapy focused on the fear and its resolution is the cornerstone of treatment.

ROLE OF THE FAMILY

Family members are critically important to the outcome of emotional problems in older adults. The first function of family members is recognition that a change has occurred in the mental status of their relative. For the clinician, the family's description of their relative's baseline functioning and the nature of the deviations from that baseline provide information essential to the diagnostic assessment. Without the clinician's guidance, however, it is difficult for family members to recognize such change, as all families have a strong emotional investment in maintenance of their structure and dynamics. Emerging symptoms may be flatly denied or they may be attributed to other factors, most commonly to "growing older." It is for this reason that the families typically bring their relatives for evaluation at times of extreme emotional distress within the family, even though symptoms may be traced back months or years. It is also common to encounter cases in which symptomatic expression is directly tied to emotional distress in the family. This idea has been heavily researched in recent years in relationship to relapse in schizophrenia (Hirsch, 1983). These studies have indicated that high levels of hostility, criticism, or overinvolvement with the patient are strong predictors of relapse and rehospitalization.

At the evaluation stage, the clinician has two roles. He must correctly diagnose the patient's problem with adequate regard given to medical, psychological, and social factors which may be responsible for the symptoms. He must also diagnose the family dynamics with regard to the timing of the presentation for evaluation, and to interplay the symptoms and the functioning of the family as a unit.

The next important role for the clinician is to help the family understand the significance of the emotional changes in their relative. Here the clinician is an educator who can provide the family with facts about treatment and prognosis. He also has a role as an interpreter of family system dynamics. As an example, consider the common case of a depressed older woman who has spent her life meeting the needs of her husband and children. In the assessment of the patient and her family, it becomes clear that the patient always had some resentment for her role in which she gave to the family but received little in return. As the changes of aging and illness reduced her strength and energy, she wished to be free of some of those expectations, but her family could not tolerate her giving up her long established role. Thus trapped and feeling hopeless, she became severely depressed. The role of the clinician at this level is to interpret the family dynamics and form an alliance with the entire family around the ideas that the entire family is in distress, and that changes in family expectations are essential to reduction of the symptoms of the patient and of the overall distress of the family.

The next step is for the clinician and the family to use the therapeutic alliance to the benefit of all. One of the most important areas of collaboration is that of medication compliance. Appropriate and judicious use of psychotropic medications can produce significant relief from the symptoms of the disorders discussed in the preceding. The clinician must educate the family as to the importance of this treatment. However, he must continually stress that medication is only a partial solution. In other words, he must confront two forms of family denial, that their relative does not have a condition which requires treatment, and that their relative's symptoms are independent of psychosocial factors and therefore must be treated with medication alone. The latter problem generally comes most clearly into focus when a family demands a medication change for increased symptomatology which the clinician sees as directly related to family dynamics.

Beyond medication, the principle therapeutic issue is to help the family understand the relationship between their older relative's symptoms and family dynamics. Some interactions are simple and straightforward. In the case of the demented patient who is easily overwhelmed by sensory stimuli and who copes poorly with environmental change, an educational approach is often all that is required. If the family members can understand their role in triggering symptoms by activities which increase environmental confusion, specific instructions on maintenance of a structured, predictable environment for their relative are generally sufficient.

For a depressed older patient, the issue of changes in the patient's family role must be addressed. Some families need help in understanding that maintenance of life-long roles is critical to the self-esteem of their older relatives, and that attempts, however well-meaning, to take over those roles may induce depression. Other families become so tied to the role of the elder that they cannot allow that person to change. Such demands, sometimes expressed even in the face of obvious, severe disability, can produce a trap from which escape seems impossible. In a more complicated case of this sort, the therapist must conduct true family therapy. Patterns of interaction among the family members must be observed and interpreted in terms of alliance and control. The significance of the patient's behavior to the equilibrium of the family must be understood by the therapist and clarified to the family. Finally, the family members must be supported through taking the necessary personal risks which will allow the patient to escape the trap.

CONCLUSION

Even the most biologically determined psychiatric illnesses such as Alzheimer's disease and schizophrenia can vary in their symptomatic presentation due to psychosocial variables. For affective and anxiety disorders, psychosocial variables can cause and maintain the symptoms. Most older adults live with one or more family members, and family dynamics are generally the most important psychosocial factors. It should be clear that some form of family intervention is necessary to properly treat an older adult with a psychiatric illness. The double barrier of resistance to working with the elderly, and resistance to dealing with families rather than individuals works against provision of optimal treatment. A clinician must maintain a strong conviction as to the necessity of such an approach or treatment will be partial at best.

REFERENCES

Bergmann, K., Foster, E.M., Justice, A.W., and Matthews, V. (1978). Management of the Demented Elderly Patient in the Community. *British Journal of Psychiatry*, 132, 441-449.

Blazer, D., and Williams, C.D. (1980). Epidemiology of Dysphoria and Depression in an Elderly Population. *American Journal of Psychiatry*, 137, 439-444.

Blessed, G., and Wilson, I.D. (1982). The Contemporary Natural History of Mental Disorder in Old Age. *British Journal of Psychiatry*, 141, 59-67.

Eisdorfer, C. (1980). Paranoia and Schizophrenic Disorders in Later Life. In:

E.W. Busse and D.G. Blazer (Eds.), *Handbook of Geriatric Psychiatry* (pp. 329-337), New York: Van Nostrand Reinhold.

Hirsch, S.R. (1983). Psychosocial Factors in the Cause and Prevention of Relapse in Schizophrenia. *British Medical Journal*, 286, 1600-1601.

Larson, E.B., Reifler, B.V., Canfield, C. and Cohen, G.D. (1984). Evaluating Elderly Outpatients With Symptoms of Dementia. *Hospital and Community Psychiatry*, 35, 425-428.

Lewis, J.M., and Johansen, K.H. (1982). Resistances to Psychotherapy With the Elderly. *American Journal of Psychotherapy*, 26, 497-504.

Rabins, P.V. (1983). Reversible Dementia and the Misdiagnosis of Dementia: A Review. *Hospital and Community Psychiatry*, 34, 830-835.

Schmidt, G.L., and Keyes, B. (1985). Group Psychotherapy with Family Caregivers of Demented Patients. *The Gerontologist*, 25, 347-350.

Weissman, M.M., Myers, J.K., Tischler, G.L., Holzer, C.E., Leaf, P.J., Orvaschel, H., and Brody, J.A. (1985). Psychiatric Disorders (DSM-III) and Cognitive Impairment Among the Elderly in a U.S. Urban Community. *Acta Psychiatrica Scandinavica*, 71, 366-379.

Caring for the Depressed Elderly and Their Families

Richard P. McQuellon
Burton V. Reifler

SUMMARY. Depression is a common problem among the elderly affecting individual patients and families as well. Even though it is a common condition, depression in the aged is undertreated due to problems in defining and diagnosing depression, the viewing of depressive symptoms as normal, and lack of a tested, integrative model of depression in the elderly. This paper addresses some of the issues facing practitioners treating depressed elderly and their families. It offers a Biopsychosocial Family-Centered Approach to comprehensive assessment illustrated with a brief case study. Several effective approaches to caring for the elderly, including somatic and non-somatic treatment interventions are described.

DEPRESSION IN THE ELDERLY

Depression is one of the most common disorders of old age, affecting a substantial number of individuals and their families. However, precise rates of depression in the elderly are unknown. One survey of elderly people living in the community reported the rate of significant depressive symptomatology at nearly 15%, including approximately 4% of the total who were suffering from a major depressive disorder (Blazer and Williams, 1980). Other surveys with special populations and using different diagnostic criteria have reported much higher rates of depressive symptoms, ranging from

---

Richard P. McQuellon, PhD, is Assistant Professor, Departments of Psychiatry & Behavioral Medicine and Family & Community Medicine; and Burton V. Reifler, MD, MPH, is Professor and Chair, Department of Psychiatry & Behavioral Medicine, at Bowman Gray School of Medicine, Wake Forest University, Winston-Salem, NC 27103.

97

25-54 percent, among older adults (Blazer, Hughes and George, 1987; Dovenmuehle, Reckless and Newman, 1970; Pfeiffer and Busse, 1973; Raymond, Michaels and Steer, 1980). Depression is a major cause of psychiatric hospitalizations in the elderly accounting for nearly half of the geriatric admissions in this age group (Gurland and Cross, 1981; Myers, Sheldon and Robinson, 1963; Redick and Taube, 1980). Depression also contributes to the suicide rate among the elderly, which is higher than that of any other age group in America (Blazer, Bachar and Manton, 1986).

The elderly depressed remain undertreated. Only one percent report receiving therapy from a trained counselor or mental health treatment by a specialist (Blazer and Williams, 1980; Boorson et al., 1986). This is unfortunate given the number of patients, families, and caregivers affected. Their numbers will increase over the next twenty years, as the ratio of Americans over 65 grows from about 1 in 10 today to approximately 1 in 7 by 2006 (Bureau of the Census, 1976). While most families can tolerate short periods of depression in their elderly members, particularly if the depressive episode is seen as a variant of normal sadness, few can sustain the energy it takes to mobilize a severely withdrawn, depressed elder.

There are a number of reasons why the depressed elderly and their families often do not receive adequate care. Among these are: problems in defining and diagnosing depression; the tendency of family members and health care providers to dismiss depressive symptoms as normal; lack of a tested integrative model of depression in the elderly; and reluctance of the elderly to seek mental health care. In this paper we discuss these issues as well as describe a comprehensive assessment and treatment approach that takes account of the medical, personal and social realities faced by the elderly and their families.

DEFINITION AND DIAGNOSIS: ISSUES AND OBSTACLES

There are problems with the definition and the diagnosis of depression. Among clinicians and nonclinicians alike, the term depression is used to describe anything from a transient mood state to clinical criteria for a major depressive episode. Klerman (1983) has described the many different meanings the term can take depending on who is using it. The neurophysiologist, pharmacologist, social worker, psychologist, psychiatrist, and mental health worker as well as nonprofessionals typically define depression differently. For example, a biological psychiatrist may see depression as primarily a problem of neurotransmission; the social worker may view depression as the product of disturbed relations, particularly in the family; the psychologist may theorize that depressed people feel the way they do because they commit errors in logic or because they have learned a sense of helplessness.

Almost all people experience depressive states characterized by feelings of sadness at one time or another. The very frequency of depressive symptoms serves to blur the distinction between the normal and abnormal feeling states we label depression. Family members and elderly patients themselves may minimize the symptoms of depression since they view them as simply "the way things are" in old age. The "old age explanation" described by Davison and Neale (1986, p.450) attributes whatever personal unhappiness the elderly may feel to some ill defined physiological process of aging — the person is depressed because they are old. Family caregivers may explain away symptoms of depression, e.g., poor concentration, insomnia, declining interests, etc. as the result of aging and not seek appropriate professional care. By invoking this explanation, clinicians may be blinded to alternative explanations and possible treatment approaches.

These definitional issues are addressed somewhat by the further development of the *Diagnostic and Statistical Manual of Mental Disorders*, Revised Edition (DSM-III-R) (American Psychiatric Association, 1987). In recognizing that depression has many subtypes, the manual proposes a number of different categories of depression. It deemphasizes age as a principal factor in the classification of depression and provides a multiaxial system for classifying psychiatric disorders. The various categories of mood disorder are described in such a way that depression in the elderly can fit into the system. Table 1 prevents the diagnostic criteria for a major depressive episode found in DSM-III-R. In general, normal periods of sadness are distinguished from a major depression by the intensity, pervasiveness, and persistence of the symptoms.

TABLE 1—
Diagnostic Criteria
for Major Depressive Episode

NOTE: A "Major Depressive Syndrome" is defined as follows in criterion A.

A. At least five of the following symptoms have been present during the same two-week period and represent a change from previous functioning; at least one of the symptoms is either (1) depressed mood, or (2) loss of interest or pleasure. (Do not include symptoms that are clearly due to a physical condition, mood-incongruent delusions or hallucinations, incoherence, or marked loosening of associations.)

(1) depressed mood (or can be irritable mood in children and adolescents) most of the day, nearly every day, as indicated either by subjective account or observation by others

(2) markedly diminished interest or pleasure in all, or almost all, activities most of the day, nearly every day (as indicated either by subjective account or observation by others of apathy most of the time)

(3) significant weight loss or weight gain when not dieting (e.g., more than 5% of body weight in a month), or decrease or increase in appetite nearly every day (in children, consider failure to make expected weight gains)

(4) insomnia or hypersomnia nearly every day

(5) psychomotor agitation or retardation nearly every day (observable by others, not merely subjective feelings of restlessness or being slowed down)

(6) fatigue or loss of energy nearly every day

(7) feelings of worthlessness or excessive or inappropriate guilt (which may be delusional) nearly every day (not merely self-reproach or guilt about being sick)

(8) diminished ability to think or concentrate, or indecisiveness, nearly every day (either by subjective account or as observed by others)

(9) recurrent thoughts of death (not just fear of dying), recurrent suicidal ideation without a specific plan, or a suicide attempt or a specific plan for committing suicide

B. (1) It cannot be established that an organic factor initiated and maintained the disturbance.

(2) The disturbance is not a normal reaction to the death of a loved one. (Uncomplicated Bereavement.)

Note: Morbid preoccupation with worthlessness, suicidal ideation, marked functional impairment or psychomotor retardation, or prolonged duration suggest bereavement complicated by Major Depression.

C. At no time during the disturbance have there been delusions or hallucinations for as long as two weeks in the absence of prominent mood symptoms (i.e., before the mood symptoms developed or after they have remitted).

D. Not superimposed on Schizophrenia, Schizophreniform Disorder, Delusional Disorder, or Psychotic Disorder NOS.

Even though clear diagnostic criteria are available there are a number of obstacles to the accurate diagnosis of depression in the elderly (Blazer and Williams, 1980; Klerman, 1983). First, manifestations of physical illness may erroneously be labeled as depression. Some common examples include hypothyroidism, pernicious anemia, uremia, congestive heart failure, and malignancies. Second, prescribed medications such as antihypertensives, antiparkinsonian agents, corticosteroids, antituberculosis medications and anticancer agents are all known to cause depression. Third, the elderly may not recognize their own symptoms or may be reluctant to report them. Fourth, clinicians may overlook mild or even severe depression that involves numerous somatic complaints. Conversely, patients with physical illness may be falsely identified as depressed since some rating scales, e.g., the Zung Self-Rating Depression Scale, weight physical symptoms heavily in the diagnosing of depressive disorder. Fifth, clinicians may too readily accept symptoms of depression in the elderly as due to old age rather than depressive illness. Finally, depression may go unrecognized when it coexists with other conditions such as dementia (Reifler, Larson and Hanley, 1982).

Clear diagnostic criteria and recognition of the various obstacles to diagnosis can aid in the clinical assessment process. Additionally, a model or a method of understanding depression is essential.

MODELS OF DEPRESSION

Like the proverbial blind men describing the elephant they feel, researchers and clinicians alike "see" different aspects of depression. Depending on their discipline, training, and theoretical vantage point, they may treat depressed patients differently. Doherty and Baird (1983) cite Usdin (1977) and suggest that causal models and treatment strategies reflect a move toward an approach that acknowledges the genetic, biochemical, psychological and social/environmental factors in depression. Such a pluralistic approach may direct clinicians to prescribe specific types of treatment with or without medication for patients with particular types of depression (Weissman, 1981). A necessary precondition for this type of treatment is a model of depression in the elderly. Here we briefly describe systemic models of depression and an integrated model of depression in the elderly.

A number of systemic models of depression have been developed by family and interpersonally oriented therapists (Coyne, 1976; Feldman, 1976; Teichman, 1986). These models are based on an understanding of family functioning through the application of systems theory (cf. Egan and Cowan, 1979; Von Bertalanffey, 1968). In its simplest form, systems theory predicts that the members of a family or system will affect and be affected by depression in one of its members. The depressed elderly patient exists in a web of disrupted relationships that can be a cause and/or a consequence of their suffering. For instance, those caregivers responsible for meeting the needs of the depressed patient may themselves become depressed (Drinka, Smith and Drinka, 1987). The likelihood of caregiver depression increases when caregivers are asked to do more than they are able to do (Litwak and Kail, 1983). All systemic models direct attention to the reciprocal influence of family and elderly identified patient.

Several authors have proposed integrative models of depression in the elderly (Breslau and Haug, 1983; Chaisson-Stewart, 1985). Breslau and Haug (1983) developed a model that is simple enough to use and complex enough to account for the reality it attempts to explain. It incorporates developmental changes, special age related vulnerabilities, and the consequences of depression in the elderly. Figure 1 illustrates the sequential nature of the model. Depression may begin with the elderly facing problems related to biological changes, increasing disability, and a sense of helplessness not encountered earlier in life. These problems, called developmental factors, are primarily bodily changes such as sensory loss. Vulnerabilities are special weaknesses in the aged, areas of function that are highly sensitive to the pressures of the aging stage of the life cycle. Examples of vulnerable areas include cognition, neurotransmission, ego function, and external support systems. Vulnerabilities often interact with precipitating events to "cause" depression. Clinical derivatives, such as helplessness behavior and social consequences

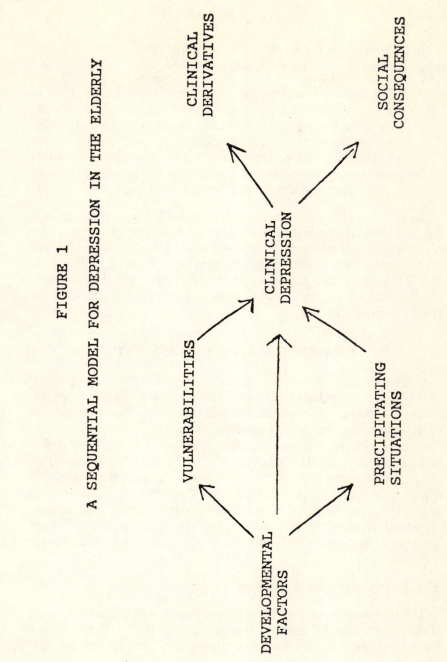

FIGURE 1

A SEQUENTIAL MODEL FOR DEPRESSION IN THE ELDERLY

such as destructive relationships with health care providers, result when depression is not satisfactorily resolved.

The model calls attention to the postulate that developmental forces challenge the adaptive system at vulnerable points. When no mastery ensues, the breakdown continues in the form of a wide range of clinical manifestations that require further identification. The entire sequence also produces nonclinical social consequences that go beyond the old person and his or her immediate environment. (Breslau and Haug, 1983, p.278)

Breslau and Haug maintain that depression is a specific disease in the aged differing from that in other age groups. Vulnerabilities, precipitating situations, clinical derivatives and social consequences of the final years are qualitatively different from those of earlier periods. Their sequential model for understanding depression provides the clinician with a useful tool for approaching the assessment of the elderly depressed.

COMPREHENSIVE ASSESSMENT

Comprehensive assessment demands sensitivity to a wide range of biological, psychological, social and spiritual issues that confront the elderly. Clear diagnostic criteria as well as causal models of depression are useful in answering the *what* and *why* of depression in the elderly. *What* are the characteristic symptoms and *why* is this patient depressed? However, as noted earlier, any number of medications, organic problems or diseases can produce depressive symptomatology. Causal models and diagnostic criteria are not enough. A broader assessment framework is necessary: the biopsychosocial approach developed by psychiatrist and internist George Engel and the concept of family centered medical care provide such a framework.

The Biopsychosocial Approach

The biopsychosocial model of medical care was formulated as an alternative to the biomedical model (Engel, 1977). It provides a framework for understanding the relationship between the biological, psychological, and social dimensions of health, disease, and health care (Doherty, Baird and Becker, 1986). Engel drew on general systems theory and proposed that the diagnostic and treatment process must account for multiple components of the patient.

The biopsychosocial model encourages a broader understanding of the elderly patient in context and helps clinicians avoid narrow conceptualization of the symptoms presented. The biological, psychological, and social dimensions of the patient can be assessed under this framework. For example, at the biological level, depression can be understood as a problem of neurochemical functioning or the result of some other physiological or disease process (Davis, Segal and Spring, 1983); at the psychological level, depression can be viewed as the product of characteristic errors in logic (Beck, 1967) or a failure to produce activities that are reinforcing (Lewinsohn, 1974); at the level of social relations, depression is seen as the result of broken attachments (Klerman et al., 1984). Of course, the biological, psychological, and social are not mutually exclusive domains. There may be impairment in each area and overlap among the three. In the depressed elderly this approach is especially useful since there are often physical, personal, and social dimensions to the patients depressed mood (Fry, 1986).

Family-Centered Medical Care

The concept of family centered medical care has been described primarily as an approach to patients for family physicians (Doherty and Baird, 1987). The concept is broadened here, since it has relevance for a wide variety of health care practitioners. There are two important elements in this approach as applied to the depressed elderly: expanded problem solving and caring for the family. First, expanding the context of problem solving beyond individual, biological dimensions may lead both the patient along with his/her family and the health care provider to a more complete understanding of depressive symptoms. Second, it is important to care for the family as well as the patient. The elderly depressed are imbedded in a psychosocial context, often family, that feels their suffering. It is these caregivers that need the help of professionals to sustain their efforts. Caring for the family is an extension of caring for the individual patient who remains at the center of the therapeutic system. Also, it is impossible to have a complete understanding of the depressed older patient without knowledge of their family context (Freeman, Epstein and Simons, 1987).

Combining the biopsychosocial approach with family-centered care of the patient can direct the clinician and family to effective interventions. For example, the patient diagnosed with depression as well as dementia of the Alzheimer's type presents a bleak picture when viewed only from a narrow, biomedical perspective. There is no cure for the degenerative process in Alzheimer's. However, the personal and social realities confronting the patient and family can be addressed. The depression can be treated with medication and/or environmental manipulation, such as enrollment in an adult day care center. These treatment strategies improve the quality of life for patient and family alike.

There is nothing new about a biopsychosocial, family-centered approach. Health care professionals have for years functioned as teams, offering multidisciplinary assessment approaches to patient care, especially in inpatient settings. The novel aspects of this approach lie in the powerful integrating capacity of the biopsychosocial model and the equal emphasis on family and patient in assessment and treatment. Biopsychosocial, family-centered care is a *way of thinking* with practical implications for working with the depressed elderly. The practical implications are seen in particular steps in the assessment process.

Practical Assessment

The steps involved in assessing a depressed elderly patient can range from a clinician conducting a single interview with the patient alone to a multidisciplinary team interviewing both patient and family and/or caregivers. It may involve psychological testing, interviews with family, and/or a home visit. While a multidisciplinary approach is not always practical it may be necessary for more complex manifestations of depression. The result of complete assessment is a clear description of the patient's symptoms, an overall understanding of the patient's problem situation, and some judgment about causal mechanisms for the depression. This process should then lead to logical treatment interventions.

There are a number of useful tools for systematically collecting diagnostic information. These include classification systems such as the DSM-III-R and psychological inventories. The DSM-III-R provides a solid descriptive system with specific criteria for mood disorders such as a major depressive syndrome. Familiarity with the various categories of mood disorder allows the clinician to classify the presenting symptoms by clinical interview.

A number of inventories have been used to assess depression in the elderly (Kaszniak and Allender, 1985). The Hamilton Rating Scale for Depression (Hamilton, 1967) is one of the most widely used instruments of this type. It is administered in interview format and highlights a number of areas such as depressed mood, feelings of guilt, suicidal thoughts, insomnia, etc. Simpler, self-administered instruments include The Beck Depression Inventory (Beck, 1967) and the Geriatric Depression Scale (GDS) (Yesavage et al., 1983). The GDS is the only instrument to date that attempts to account for the unique problem encountered when diagnosing depression in the elderly, such as the increased number of somatic complaints in this population.

Interviews with the patient and caregivers and/or family members as well can provide an overall picture of social functioning and qualitative aspects of the patient's life. Constructing a visual portrayal of the family, called a genogram, provides a general picture of the family system and clues to symptom clusters that make their way across generations (McGoldrick and Gerson, 1985). Since the patient's living situation and social context may not be depicted in the genogram, it is important to gather information about the patient's immediate living environment and broader social network including involvement in church, civic, neighborhood and living group activities. A person isolated from family, friendship or living community ties is at risk for dyphoria if not an episode of major depressive disorder.

The elderly frequently suffer from chronic illness requiring continued medical management and drug therapy. Organic disease, such as hypothyroidism, and any number of medications (cf. Spar, 1985) can produce depressive symptoms. A thorough review of medical problems, lab tests where indicated, and a complete drug inventory are necessary to differentiate depressions of primary or secondary origin.

Family-centered, biopsychosocial assessment makes use of information supplied by the patient and his/her family. This information can then be synthesized into hypotheses about causal mechanisms leading to appropriate treatment. For example, changing medications for hypertension when the patient has been taking one known to cause secondary depressions may produce immediate symptom relief. Simple, effective treatment approaches are probably the exception rather than the rule given the many developmental vulnerabilities facing the elderly. Nevertheless, simple as well as multidemensional causes of depression should be examined in a comprehensive assessment process.

CARING FOR THE DEPRESSED ELDERLY

A number of somatic and non-somatic treatment approaches administered individually or in combination have been found to be effective with this population. We expect that these will increase as the elderly are included in more research projects. Somatic treatment approaches include psychopharmocotherapy and ECT. (We do not include here nutritional therapies or therapies aimed at treating secondary depression that may be due to drug usage or other medical or psychiatric disorders.)

Somatic Treatment Approaches

Therapy with antidepressant medications is a consideration for elderly depressed patients, particularly in cases where the depression is chronic, where it is so severe as to be debilitating, or where the patient is very somatically oriented and resistant to psychotherapy. In some individuals, frequent recurrences of depression interfere substantially with daily living, and when psychotherapy does not seem to help, maintenance therapy with an antidepressant can often reduce the periods of disability.

When depression is so severe as to be life threatening, inpatient treatment by a psychiatrist is warranted and antidepressant medications would usually be indicated. Despite an element of public sentiment against it, electroconvulsive therapy (ETC) is safe and highly effective for severe, drug resistant depression especially when accompanied by suicidal and/or psychiatric symptoms; it is now given in carefully controlled circumstances with the aid of an anesthesiologist and carries very little risk.

With careful monitoring and use of the lowest effective dosage, antidepressant therapy can be a valuable treatment approach even in the very old. The general rule is to start low, and be prepared to slowly increase the dose if necessary. The choice of a specific antidepressant depends on elements such as history of previous success with a given agent, and the side effects of the particular drug. For example, doxepin (Sinequan, Adapin) has some sedating effects and can be used at nighttime in a depressed patient with insomnia, while desipramine (Norpramin) is activating and can be taken in the morning by a patient who is sleeping excessively during the day. A number of references provide useful guidelines for the clinician treating the depressed elderly patient on antidepressants (cf. Bowden and Giffen, 1987; Fry, 1986).

Family members of the depressed patient can be instrumental in the treatment process with antidepressants. Their support can increase adherence to the medication regimen. They can monitor and discuss side effects with the patient, clarify expectations of the medication when necessary and report progress to the patient and the patient's physician.

Non-somatic Treatment Approaches

Research on the effectiveness of psychological intervention with the elderly has been limited due to their frequent exclusion from controlled studies and pessimism about the value of therapy for this population. Additionally, the elderly are often reluctant to seek mental health care (Chaisson-Stewart, 1985) and may be victims of funding discrimination against the aged and mentally ill (Larson and Reifler, 1987). However, there is a growing body of literature supporting the efficacy of psychological intervention for older adults (Gatz, Popkin, Pino and VandenBos, 1985). Especially helpful for the elderly depressed, are the interpersonal and cognitive-behavioral approaches (Fry, 1986). Here we cite two representative studies from the literature:

Gallagher and Thompson (1983) studied the effectiveness of psychotherapy for both endogenous and non-endogenous depression in adults age 55 and older. All patients were in a current episode of major depressive disorder, with half presenting with endogenous symptoms as well. The patients were treated in either behavioral, cognitive, or insight oriented psychotherapy for 16 sessions over a 12 week period. While patients categorized as non-endogenous responded more favorably to psychotherapy, significant improvement was also made by some endogenous patients. The authors conclude that their results support psychotherapy as effective with older adults, especially for those patients who cannot or will not take psychotropic medications for depression.

Sholomskas et al. (1983), reported positive case study results from a pilot project designed to test the efficacy of Interpersonal Psychotherapy (IPT) with ambulatory outpatients over age 60 who met Research Diagnostic Criteria (RDC) and DSM-III criteria for major depression. The IPT model emphasizes the processes between people that may be disrupted in four specific areas: Grief, interpersonal disputes, role transitions, and interpersonal deficits. In this study, the therapist took an active, collaborative, patient advocate role. The initial sessions were used to elicit the history of the depressive condition, to learn of the patient's significant interpersonal relationships and to set treatment goals. In subsequent sessions, the task was to guide the patient to cover material related to the goals. From their generally positive experience with these cases, the authors suggest specific considerations in psychotherapy with the elderly. These include: an active therapeutic stance by the therapist; flexibility in session length; recognition of the patient's increased dependency needs; attention to social and environmental problems; and tolerance by the therapist for necessary limitations on therapy such as unsolvable social problems, long-standing pathology and maladaptation and the questions of meaning and purpose facing the aged.

Both studies noted here describe interventions with individuals, even though the interpersonal approach emphasizes between-people processes that affect mood. Family-centered treatment approaches with the elderly are not well represented in the literature, and few conclusions can be made about their efficacy. However, Fry (1987, p.385) suggests that family ties do not diminish with age, and may play an increasing role in sustaining elderly who have diminished social support systems. It remains the promise of family-centered therapists to provide tested therapeutic procedures necessary for helping families respond to their depressed elders. The clinical efficacy of a biopsychosocial, family-centered treatment approach is illustrated in the following case study.

THE CASE OF MRS. B.

Mrs. B. is an 83-year-old white, divorced, female who lives with Bob, her common law husband of 10 years. She was referred for therapy by her family physician and presented with the following symptoms: difficulty falling asleep and early morning awakening, loss of interest in daily activities, depressed mood which she described as worse in the morning, irritability, and fatigue. Her major complaints centered around four areas. First, she suffered numerous health problems including angina, osteoarthritis of the knees, and correctable loss in hearing and sight. Second, she described frequent verbal conflict with Bob noting that he drank heavily and frequently denigrated her. Third, she had recently discontinued her hospital volunteer work due to changes in parking policy making the walk from the lot to the hospital too difficult for her. Finally, she feared that her current symptoms would develop into an incapacitating depression.

Mrs. B. described a history of 7-8 episodes of serious depression dating back to 1945. Her mother, who committed suicide, and grandmother also suffered from depression. She had been treated with ECT, various medications, and psychotherapy during these periods which usually resolved within 2 to 3 months. Most recently she had been treated with Lithobid, 300 mg/day for manic depressive illness, depressed type, initially started by her psychiatrist and maintained by her family physician. Her last inpatient care had been for several weeks 8 years ago.

Mrs. B.'s social resources included her son and daughter-in-law who lived nearby and provided instrumental and emotional support.

She spoke weekly with a second married son who lived in a distant city. Her dog, Tulip, was a source of love and companionship. She was minimally involved in community activities and did not attend church.

The initial treatment plan consisted of: (1) weekly, supportive, problem solving counseling designed to address the loss of volunteer work and conflict with Bob; (2) referral to Al-Anon; (3) encouragement to pursue volunteer work; (4) family assessment through a home visit; (5) consultation between her family physician and psychologist provided for continuity of care.

Her depressive symptoms were partially relieved in approximately 3 months and she became less frightened of slipping into a major depression. Even though she had some symptomatic relief, she was unable to make any changes in her relationship with Bob and continued to be distressed by her physical ailments. She did not attend Al-Anon but reported that Bob had stopped drinking following an auto accident where he was arrested for driving under the influence of alcohol. She became involved in volunteer work again at another location and has continued in follow-up supportive counseling every 4-6 weeks.

This case illustrates a number of the issues raised in the assessment and treatment of the depressed elderly. First, it is important to utilize several causal models of depression to understand the patient's situation. By family history and previous treatment, Mrs. B. suffered from recurrent episodes of debilitating depression, diagnosed as manic depressive illness, depressed type. There were genetic and biochemical components to her distress. Yet, she was not experiencing a bout of major depression — she feared it would develop from her situational stressors, i.e., conflict with Bob, nagging health problems, and loss of meaningful volunteer work. The source of her sadness was in these areas, and required treatment of interpersonal disputes and role transition as well as recognition of inevitable physical decline. Second, Breslau and Haug's integrative model of depression emphasizes the developmental changes confronting the elderly. Mrs. B. faced increasing disability and a sense of helplessness when institutional parking changes made it difficult for her to continue volunteer work. This precipitating situation forced more conflicted interaction with Bob and highlighted the physical and emotional vulnerabilities of her aging. Third, a bio-psychosocial, family-centered approach provided a powerful conceptualization of Mrs. B.'s situation. She had numerous physical ailments treated by her family physician who also managed her medications, and maintained periodic contact with the patient's son and therapist. The therapist spoke with family members including Bob, and conducted a home visit, which provided insight into the patient's relationship with Bob and her dog, Tulip. Finally, the caring relationship provided by the family physician and therapist was a source of comfort and a new support system that Mrs. B. could draw upon for help.

CONCLUSION

Depression affects a significant number of the elderly and their families as well. It is frequently referred to as "one of the most common disorders of old age." While common, it is not the result of normal aging. The inevitable losses which accompany the aging process do not necessarily lead to clinical depression. Depression in the elderly should and can be treated effectively with a number of methods.

There are numerous definitional issues and diagnostic obstacles to the accurate assessment of depression. Refinements in diagnostic criteria noted in the DMS-III-R and further development of instruments such as the Geriatric Depression Scale contribute to a more precise definition of depression in the elderly. Recognition of the obstacles to accurate diagnosis, such as physical illnesses which produce depressive symptoms, serve to alert clinicians to the hazards of applying narrow causal models in the assessment process.

Systemic and interpersonal models of depression are especially useful with the elderly who may suffer from a sense of isolation and loneliness. These models can be nested in the biopsychosocial, family-centered approach to comprehensive assessment. This approach emphasizes the complex interplay among the biological, psychological, and social dimensions of patients and the necessity for family involvement in the assessment and treatment process. Somatic and non-somatic treatment regimens, alone or combined, have been effective with the elderly depressed. Family-centered treatment approaches hold the potential for releasing the healing properties in family ties. They hold much promise and have yet to be fully utilized or researched.

REFERENCES

American Psychiatric Association. (1987). Diagnostic and statistical manual of mental disorders. (Third edition, revised.) Washington, D.C.: American Psychiatric Association.

Beck, A.T. (1967). Depression: Clinical, experimental and theoretical aspects. New York: Harper and Row.

Blazer, D., Hughes, D.C., and George, L.K., (1987). The Epidemiology of depression in an elderly community population. The Gerontologist, 27, 281-287.

Blazer, D., and Williams, C.D. (1980). Epidemiology of dysphoria and depression in an elderly population. American Journal of Psychiatry, 137, 439-444.

Blazer, D.G., Bachar, J.R., and Manton, K.G. (1986). Suicide in late life: Review and commentary. Journal of the American Geriatric Society, 34, 519-525.

Boorson, S., Barnes, R.A., Kukull, W.A., Okinioto, J.T., Veith, R.C., Inui, T.S., Carter, W., and Raskind, M. (1986). Symptomatic depression in elderly medical outpatients: I. Prevalence, demography, and health service utilization. Journal of the American Geriatric Society, 34, 341-347.

Bowden, C.L., and Giffen, M.B. (1987). Psychopharmacology for Primary Care Physicians. (Second edition.) Baltimore: Williams and Wilkins.

Breslau, L.D., and Haug, M.R. (1983). Some elements in an integrative model of depression in the aged. In L.D. Breslau and M.R. Haug (Eds.), Depression and Aging: causes, care, and consequences. New York: Springer.

Bureau of the Census (1976). Demographic aspects of aging and the older population in the United States. Current Population Reports: Special Studies, Series 23, No.59. Washington, D.C.: U.S. Government Printing Office.

Chaisson-Stewart, G.M. (1985). An integrated theory of depression. In G.M. Chaisson-Stewart (Ed.), Depression in the elderly: An interdisciplinary approach. New York: John Wiley.

Chaisson-Stewart, G.M. (1985). Tragedies of inappropriate or inadequate treatment. In G.M. Chaisson-Stewart (Ed.), Depression in the elderly: An interdisciplinary approach. New York: John Wiley.

Coyne, J.C. (1976). Toward an interactional description of depression. Psychiatry, 39, 28-40.

Davis, J.M., Segal, N.L., and Spring, G.K. (1983). Biological and genetic aspects of depression in the elderly. In L.D. Breslau and M.R. Haug (Eds.), Depression and aging: Causes, care and consequences. New York: Springer.

Davison, G.C., and Neale, J.M. (1986). Abnormal psychology: An experimental clinical approach. (4th Ed.), New York: John Wiley.

Doherty, W.J., and Baird, M.A. (1983). Family therapy and family medicine: Toward the primary care of families. New York: Guilford Press.

Doherty, W.J., and Baird, M.A. (1987). Family-centered medical care: A clinical casebook. New York: Guilford Press.

Doherty, W.J., Baird, M.A., and Becker, L.A. (1986). Family medicine as a biopsychosocial discipline: The road toward integration. In W.J. Doherty, C.E. Christianson, and M. Sussman (Eds.), Family medicine: The maturing of a discipline. New York: The Haworth Press, Inc.

Dovenmuehle, R.H., Reckless, J.B., and Newman, G. (1970). Depressive reactions in the elderly. In Normal aging: Reports from the Duke Longitudinal Study, 1955-1969. E. Palmer (Ed.), Durham, N.C.: Duke University Press.

Drinka, T.J.K., Smith, J.C., and Drinka, P.J. (1987). Correlates of depression and burden for informal caregivers of patients in a geriatrics referral clinic. Journal of the American Geriatric Society, 35, 522-525.

Egan, G., and Cowan, M.A. (1979). People in systems: A model for development in the human-service professions and education. Monterey: Brooks/Cole.

Engel, G.L. (1977). The need for a new medical model: A challenge for biomedicine. Science, 196, 129-136.

Feldman, L.B. (1976). Depression and marital interaction. Family Process, 15, 389-395.

Freeman, A., Epstein, N., and Simon, K.M. (1987). The treatment of depression in the family context: A synthesis. Journal of Psychotherapy and the Family, 314, 173-181.

Fry, P.S. (1986). Depression, stress, and adaptations in the elderly: Psychological assessment and intervention. Rockville, Md.: Aspen Publishers.

Gallagher, D.E., and Thompson, L.W. (1983). Effectiveness of psychotherapy for both endogenous and non endogenous depression in older adult outpatients. Journal of Gerontology, 38, 707-712.

Gatz, M., Popkin, S.J., Pino, C.D., and VandenBos, G.R. (1985). Psychological interventions with older adults. In J.E. Birren and K.W. Schae (Eds.) Handbook of the psychology of aging (2nd Ed.). New York: VanNostrand Reinhold.

Gurland, B.J., and Cross, P.S. (1982). Epidemiology of psychopathology in old age. In L.F. Jarvik and G.W. Small (Eds.), Psychiatric Clinics of North America. Philadelphia: Saunders.

Hamilton, M. (1967). Development of a rating scale for primary depressive illness. British Journal of Social and Clinical Psychology, 6, 278-296.

Kaszniak, A.W., and Allender, J. (1985). Psychological assessment of depression in older adults. In G.M. Chaisson-Stewart (Ed.), Depression in the elderly: An interdisciplinary approach. New York: John Wiley.

Klerman, G. (1983). Problems in the definition and diagnosis of depression in the elderly. In L.D. Breslau and M.R. Haug (Eds.), Depression and aging: Causes, care, and consequences. New York: Springer.

Klerman, G., Weissman, M.M., Rounsaville, B.J., and Chevron, E.S. (1984). Interpersonal psychotherapy of depression. New York: Basic Books.

Lewinsohn, P.H. (1974). A behavioral approach to depression. In R.J. Friedman and M.M. Katz (Eds.), The psychology of depression: Contemporary Theory and Research. Washington, D.C.: Winston: Wiley.

Litwak, E., and Kail, B. (1983). Some social costs to primary group helpers of aged depressives. In L.D. Breslau and M.R. Haug (Eds.), Depression and aging: Causes, care, and consequences. New York: Springer.

McGoldrick, M., and Gerson, R. (1985). Genograms in family assessment. New York: Norton.

Myers, J.M., Sheldon, D., and Robinson, S.S. (1963). A study of 138 elderly first admissions. American Journal of Psychiatry, 120, 244-249.

Pfeiffer, E., and Busse, E.W. (1973). Mental disorders in later life — Affective disorders: Paranoid, neurotic and situational reactions. In E.W. Busse and E. Pfeiffer (Eds.), Mental illness in later life. Washington, D.C.: American Psychiatric Association.

Raymond, E.F., Michaels, T.J., and Steer, R.A. (1980). Prevalence and correlates of depression in elderly persons. Psychological Reports, 47, 1055-1061.

Redick, R.W., and Taube, C.A. (1980). Demography and mental health care of the aged. In J.E. Birren and R. B. Sloane (Eds.), Handbook of mental health and aging. Englewood Cliffs, N.J.: Prentice Hall.

Reifler, B.V., and Larson, E. (1988). Excess disability in dementia of the Alzheimers type. In E. Light and B. Lebowitz (Eds.), Alzheimers disease treatment and family stress: Directions for research. Washington, D.C.: Printing Office.

Reifler, B.V., Larson, E., and Hanley, R. (1982). Coexistence of cognitive impairment and depression in geriatric outpatients. American Journal of Psychiatry, 139, 623-626.

Sholomskas, A.J., Chevron, E.S., Prusoff, B.A., and Berry, C. (1983). Short-term interpersonal therapy (IPT) with the depressed elderly: case reports and discussion. American Journal of Psychotherapy, 37, 552-566.

Spar, J.E. (1985). Drug treatment. In G.M. Chaisson-Stewart (Ed.), Depression in the elderly: An interdisciplinary approach. New York: John Wiley.

Teichman, Y. (1986). Family therapy of depression. Journal of Psychotherapy and the Family, 3/4, 9-39.

Usdin, G. (1977). Introduction. In G. Usdin (Ed.), Depression: Clinical, biological, and psychological perspectives. New York: Brunner/Mazel.

Von Bertalanffey, L.A. (1986). General systems theory (Rev. Ed.). New York: Braziller.

Yesavage, J.A., Brink, T.L., Rose, T.L., Lum, O., Huang, V., Adey, M., and Leirer, V. (1983). Development and validation of a geriatric depression screening scale: A preliminary report. Journal of Psychiatric Research, 17, 37-49.

A Systems Approach
to Suicide Prevention

Nancy J. Osgood

SUMMARY. The paper explores various factors contributing to suicide among the elderly; outlines major theoretical and conceptual models which are relevant to the issues; and highlights techniques of assessing suicide risk and strategies of preventing suicide among the elderly. Clues and warning signs of late life suicide are presented. The important role of the family in suicide and suicide prevention is discussed in depth. The role of the practitioner in working with the "at risk" individual and his/her family is also discussed in detail.

INTRODUCTION

The people most "at risk" for suicide are the elderly. Their suicide rate is 50 percent higher than that of the young. In 1983 U.S. suicide rates were 12.1 per 100,000 for the nation, 11.9 for those 15 to 24 years old, and 19.2 for those 65 and over (NCHS, 1985). In spite of these statistics, most attention has focused on young people; until recently the problem of suicide among the old has virtually been ignored. Although the act of suicide is an individual act, suicide occurs in the social context of the family system. To date, very little attention has been paid to the family system as a causal factor in suicidal behavior or as a factor in the prevention of such behavior.

In this article suicide among the elderly will be explored in terms of contributing factors, theoretical explanations, and conceptual models. Assessment of suicidal risk and suicide prevention techniques and strategies will also be discussed. The role of family members in suicide detection and prevention will be highlighted.

Nancy J. Osgood, PhD, is Associate Professor, Gerontology and Sociology, Medical College of Virginia, Richmond, VA.

Finally, the role of the practitioner in working with "at risk" elders and their families will be emphasized.

DEMOGRAPHIC FACTORS IN GERIATRIC SUICIDE

Certain segments of the elderly population are more likely than others to commit suicide. Age, gender, and race are important demographic variables. The "old old" (75+) are at greatest risk of committing suicide (McIntosh, 1984; Kastenbaum, 1985).

Particularly at risk are elderly white males. The suicide rate for white females peaks in mid-life and then declines, whereas the male suicide rate continues to increase through the eighth decade (Miller, 1979). The ratio of male to female suicides in the 65-69 age group is about 4:1, compared to a ratio of 12:1 by age 85 (Miller, 1979).

A similar situation exists with respect to suicide among whites and nonwhites. The trend for whites is an increase in suicides through the last stages of the life cycle. By contrast, minority suicide rates peak between 25 and 30 years of age and then decline through the late years (McIntosh, 1985).

Unmarried elderly are more likely than married to commit suicide, elderly widowers being the most vulnerable (Berardo, 1970). Elderly living in urban areas, particularly low-income transient areas in central cities, are more "at risk" than are those living in rural areas (Sainsbury, 1963). The elderly living alone also are at greater risk (Gubrium, 1974).

THEORETICAL EXPLANATIONS
AND CONCEPTUAL MODELS

Several cultural, social, and psychological explanations for the higher rate of suicide among the elderly have been offered. The cultural explanation posits a strong relationship between level of modernization (based on level of technology, degree of urbanization, rate of social change, and degree of westernization) and status of the elderly. In western technologically advanced societies such as ours the elderly are devalued and hold less power, status, and economic control than in less advanced societies. In such a society the knowledge and wisdom of elders is not recognized or respected.

Older adults are viewed as useless, nonproductive, and obsolete — a burden to be borne by younger members. In such a culture the old lose status and their self-concept suffers. They may see no sense of meaning and purpose in life and feel devalued, unloved, unneeded and unwanted. Suicide may represent a personal expression of their reaction to negative cultural images.

Various sociological explanations of the high rate of elderly suicide exist. In his famous work, *Suicide*, Emile Durkheim (1951) proposed that suicide increased with age because society as a moral force begins to recede from the person in terms of both goals and commitments, as the person ages and withdraws from various roles and positions, becoming less integrated into and less dependent upon society. Building on the early work of Durkheim, Rosow (1967) suggested that the elderly tend to be less integrated into society because of (1) their removal and withdrawal from certain organizational contexts and associated roles, with resultant weakening of ties to mediating structures, such as work, voluntary associations, and like organizations; and (2) the contraction of their intimate social world as a result of relocation, incapacitation, and death of friends and peers.

Those employing sociologial models have explained the higher suicide rate for elderly white males as a function of greater social loss. Compared to women and minority males in our society, elderly white males suffer the most severe loss of social roles, status, power and money (McIntosh and Santos, 1981), resulting in greater loss of identity and self-esteem. Compared to elderly blacks, elderly whites are less likely to find support in their families, church, and community. Seiden (1981) argues that elderly blacks are wanted and needed in the family system, sometimes because of economic necessity but also because old age is respected by blacks, who feel that elders belong and are useful and productive.

Psychological explanations for the high rate of suicide among the elderly have predominated in the literature. In his early work Freud (1917) contended that loss of a loved one results in feelings of abandonment and rejection, which may swell into anger directed against the lost loved one. Loss results in a particular state of mind in the individual. In an attempt to kill the memory of the lost loved one, suicide may result. Influenced by Freud's earlier work, several psychological explanations of suicide have focused on the concepts of loss and depression as they affect the state of mind of the individual and perhaps induce suicide.

Many older persons lose vital social roles in the world of work, family, politics, and community. In addition, many also suffer physical losses — declining health, painful chronic debilitating illness, loss of a limb, hearing, or eyesight — that they find almost impossible to bear. Others experience deep personal losses, such as the death of a spouse or close friend.

Multiple losses in rapid succession often accompany the aging process. These losses can result in increased stress for the older individual at a time when he/she is most vulnerable and least resistant to stress. According to Mary Miller (1979) "whether an older person is able to resolve a suicidal crisis or succumbs to self-inflicted death is very much a function of the ability to cope with stress." Loss and stress can result in loneliness, alcoholism, hopelessness, depression, and despair. Depression and alcoholism have been identified as major factors in late life suicide.

Depression, the most common functional psychiatric disorder of late life, underlies two-thirds of the suicides in the elderly (Gurland and Cross, 1983). Three major factors have been recognized as contributing to depression and suicide among the aged: haplessness, helplessness, and hopelessness. The aged are most susceptible to helplessness, according to Seligman (1975), because they have experienced the greatest loss of control. Karl Menninger (1938) characterized suicides of the elderly as a result of the wish to die, emphasizing hopelessness as a major factor. Analysis of suicide notes (Cath, 1965; Farberow and Shneidman, 1970) left by older adults have revealed a sense of "psychological exhaustion," a tiredness of living.

Alcoholism is another major factor in geriatric suicide. Blazer (1982) points out that the relationship between alcoholism and suicide is greatest in late life. To relieve depression and loneliness and escape from the multiple problems and stresses of growing old, many turn to alcohol. Instead of relieving depression, ingesting large quantities of alcohol actually increases depression and anxiety. Alcohol acts as a depressant on the central nervous system and may also alter moods and decrease critical life-evaluating functions of the ego, allowing unconscious self-destructive impulses to gain control. The stimulating effects of alcohol may reduce inhibitions and self-control and contribute to the "courage" some feel is a factor in suicide. Continued regular use of alcohol often results in the deterioration of important social relationships, primarily in the family and among friends, leading to social alienation and isolation. Anger, hostility, and belligerence associated with frequent drinking alienate family members and close friends at the time when the depressed elderly drinker most needs social and emotional support. Coupled with increased social isolation and alienation are intense feelings of shame, guilt, denial, pessimism, and lower self-concept, all factors in suicidal behavior.

ASSESSMENT OF SUICIDAL RISK

Because of the importance of depression and alcoholism as factors in geriatric suicide, recognition of the existence of either or both of these conditions is crucial to assessment of suicidal risk.

In the elderly, depression often manifests itself in specific somatic complaints, including changes in eating and sleeping patterns, fatigue, increased heart rate, headaches and muscle pains, constipation, and other concerns with bodily functions. Depressed elderly persons are anxious, preoccupied with physical symptoms, fatigued, withdrawn, retarded, apathetic, inert, disinterested in their surroundings, and lacking in drive. Apathy, withdrawal, and functional slowness are also common symptoms of depression in the elderly.

Warning signs of alcoholism in the elderly are similar to the signs for other age groups. Some common signs include: early morning drinking; blackouts; flushed face; tremors; behavior manifestations of anger, hostility, and belligerence; and problems with family and friends, the law, or finances related to alcohol use.

Many elderly give clues to their impending suicidal behavior. Reading these clues accurately may help save a life. Direct verbal clues include such statements as "I am going to kill myself," "I'm going to commit suicide," and "I want to end it all." Direct suicidal threats should always be taken seriously. Suicidal ideations and fantasies should also be regarded as serious clues to suicide.

Indirect verbal clues are such statements as "I'm tired of life," "What's the point of going on," and "Who cares if I'm dead anyway."

The most direct behavior clue is, of course, a suicide attempt. Indirect behavioral clues include: donating one's body to a medical school; purchasing a gun; stockpiling pills; putting personal and business affairs in order; making or changing a will; taking out insurance or changing beneficiaries; making funeral plans; giving away money and possessions; changes in behavior, especially episodes of screaming, hitting, or throwing things or failure to get along with family, friends, or peers; inability to perform various household or social tasks.

In some cases the situation itself may be the clue to suicide in the elderly. A recent move; death of a spouse, child, or friend; or diagnosis of terminal illness may precipitate a suicidal crisis in the elderly. The chart that follows provides an overview of important clues and warning signs of suicide in the elderly.

Clues and Warning Signs of Suicide in the Elderly

Verbal Clues

- I am going to kill myself.
- I'm going to commit suicide.
- I'm going to end it all.
- I want to end it all.
- I just want out.
- You would be better off without me.

Behavioral Clues

- donating body to a medical school
- purchasing a gun
- stockpiling pills
- putting personal and business affairs in order
- making or changing a will
- taking out insurance or changing beneficiaries
- making funeral plans
- giving away money and/or possessions
- changes in behavior, especially episodes of screaming or hitting, throwing things or failure to get along with family, friends or peers
- suspicious behavior, for example, going out at odd times of the day or night, waving or kissing goodbye (if not characteristic)

• sudden interest or disinterest in church and religion
• scheduling of appointment with doctor for no apparent physical cause or very shortly after the last visit to the doctor
• loss of physical skills, general confusion, or loss of understanding, judgement, or memory

Situational Clues

• recent move
• death of a spouse
• diagnosis of terminal illness
• flare-up with relative or close friend

Symptoms of Late Life Depression

• Change in sleep patterns, particularly insomnia
• Change in eating patterns, especially loss of appetite
• Weight loss
• Extreme fatigue
• Increased concern with bodily functions (e.g., frequent complaints of constipation, loose bowels, aches and pains, dizziness, increased heart rate)
• Change in mood, particularly if listless, apathetic, angry, hostile, nervous, irritable, depressed, sad, or withdrawn
• Expression of fears and anxieties without any reason
• Low self-esteem or self-concept, feelings of worthlessness, pessimism

Warning Signs of Alcoholism in the Elderly

• Increase in amount of alcohol or number of alcoholic drinks taken
• Behavioral manifestations of anger, hostility, belligerence
• Odor of alcohol on breath, especially in the morning
• Flushed face
• Trembling and the "shakes"
• Blackout periods
• Hangovers
• Alcoholic hepatitis, cirrhosis, chronic gastritis
• Drinking in spite of medical admonitions against alcohol use
• Problems with family members, friends, or relatives
• Inability to do simple tasks, confusion, slurred speech, or retarded motor skills
• Inability to conduct normal everyday tasks without drinking
• Financial problems related to alcohol use

THE ROLE OF THE FAMILY

Every individual is a member of a family. The family institution has existed as long as the human species. In an early statement on the family system Ackerman (1958) described the family as made up of a fusion of four factors: biological, psychological, social, and economic. Biologically, the family is the unit of procreation and also assures the survival of members. Psychologically, members are bound by mutual interdependence and need to satisfy affectional needs. Economically, the family provides for the satisfaction of economic and other material needs. The social purposes include "provision of food and shelter, social togetherness, companionship, the opportunity to evolve a personal and family identity, and support for individual creativity and initiative" (p. 19).

Like all systems, the family has particular goals, tasks, and functions. It encompasses levels of authority, a power structure, reciprocal role relationships, and mutual expectations. "The hierarchical organization of family includes members dominating, taking responsibility, and making decisions for others. It also includes helping, protecting, comforting, rewarding, and taking care of others" (Madanes, 1981, p. 223). The family is held together by bonds of love and affection. The major function of the family is to provide companionship among members, physical necessities, maintenance of motivation and morale, and continuing communication and patterns of interaction (Murray et al., 1980).

Family systems theory examines how family members influence and are influenced by one another. This systems view has arisen in the past 25 years. Early work with problem adolescents and their families and with schizophrenic patients and their families provided the impetus for the family therapy movement. Family therapists focus on the family system as the root of problematic behavior of any individual member and advocate work with the family system to solve the problem.

In 1965 Shanas and Streib published an important collection of writings reaffirming the importance of the family to elders and pointing out that elders need to be viewed in the social context of their family (Herr and Weakland, 1979). Since that time numerous geropsychologists, social workers, and others who counsel elders have recognized the numerous benefits of family therapy for older adults who suffer from depression and other age-related problems (Brody, 1966; Brody and Spark, 1966; Gottesman et al., 1973).

Savitsky and Sharkey (1972) argue strongly for a family systems approach to the treatment of psychological problems of elders. As they write:

> Family interaction constitutes a significant form of personal relationships in the aged. This applies not only to the individual in his active participation in the family life but also to an assessment of fluctuations in chronic, medical, and neuro-psychiatric disorders and of facts involved in the precipitation of acute disturbances. Exploration of the "family" context, utilization of family interviews, and work with individual family members are essential factors in the diagnosis and management of disturbed behavior. Exploration and interpretation of family . . . patterns constitutes significant components of staff orientation in institutional and extramural practice. (p. 19)

Viewed from this perspective the family is seen as the basic unit of health and illness. The breakdown of individuals must be viewed within the social context of the family. There is a direct relationship between the individual state of mental health and the degree of health of the family. Suicidal behavior may be an expression of family conflict and may reflect disharmony and disequilibrium in the family system. The family may be viewed as the major source of stress.

Just as the family system may be at the root of the disturbed individual's problem, it is also just as likely to be the individual's major source of strength and primary defense against the problems and crises of daily living. According to Bengtson and Treas (1980), families contribute to the mental health and well-being of members in two important ways: first, by providing a support system which offers love and affection, financial assistance, needed services, assistance with tasks, and other forms of strength and help; and secondly, influencing self-concept through social interactions, communication, and evaluations of role performance.

The elderly are particularly dependent on the family for support.

Weiss (1976) notes that support is especially important in times of crisis, transition, and stress. Many older adults face the transition to widowhood or retirement. Others face the loss of physical health and mobility or income, status, and power. Family support in the form of love and understanding, caring and concern, affection and companionship, financial assistance, and acceptance is vital to the older individual. The family can aid the older member by "helping him/her to mature; become more adaptive, integrated, and open to his/her experiences; and to find meaning in his/her situation" (Murray et al., 1980, p. 52). The family, according to Caplan (1976), functions as a collector and disseminator of information, a feedback guidance system, a source of ideology, a guide and mediator in problem solving, a source of mutual aid, a haven for rest and recuperation, a reference and control group, a source and validator of identity, and a place for emotional expression. As such, the family represents the major force for mediating the negative effects of stress and loss on older individuals.

Family members have a major role in assessing and preventing suicide in the elderly. Family members must become more aware of the demographic characteristics of the most "at risk" elderly. They should also become "depression conscious," learning to recognize the signs and symptoms of late life depression in their loved ones. They need to become more familiar with the clues and warning signs which signal suicidal intent to the elderly. Finally, family members need to carefully listen to the communications of their elderly loved one rather than tuning such cues out, ignoring the problem, and refusing to really "hear" their older relative.

Family members should be sensitive to the particular losses, stresses, and transitions facing their older relatives. Older individuals often must become the receiver of services and support rather than the provider. Families need to be willing to re-align roles and power structures to accommodate the changing needs of an older member. When a problem is apparent, families need to mobilize their energies and become self-healing groups, providing additional support in the form of love and concern, affection, acceptance, respect, and positive affirmations of the dignity and worth of the older member who is hurting. Finally, family members must be able to recognize when the problem is too serious to be handled in the context of the family alone and must be willing to seek out professional help.

SUICIDE PREVENTION

Richman (1986) suggests that before suicidal resolution of a problem occurs, four factors must be present: (1) exhaustion of the resources of the self, which occurs when the individual has suffered many deep personal and social losses over time and reached a state of hopelessness until he cries "Enough"; (2) exhaustion of the resources of the family, in which energies are spent and the family can no longer provide needed help and emotional support to the suicidal member; (3) a stage of intolerable stress, when there is a crisis that seems insoluble to everyone; and (4) the acceptance of suicide as a viable solution to life's problems on the part of the individual and other family members.

The importance of family therapy in suicide prevention cannot be overemphasized. According to Richman (1986), the major goal of family therapy is to release the healing forces each family possesses and help the family become a self-help group. The role of the therapist is a catalyst who functions to remove barriers to continued growth and development, individuation, caring, and cohesion. Herr and Weakland (1979) advocate a similar approach in which the family therapist works with troubled family members to identify and define the problem; decide on solutions and set realistic family goals; and mobilize the family system to solve the problem and reach the goals set.

According to Blazer (1982), the therapist working with families who have a depressed elderly member must evaluate the following elements of the family system: past and present psychological state of individual family members; family structure, including location, roles, and boundaries; type, quantity, and quality of interactions; family atmosphere or "ambience"; family values, especially values regarding mental health and the role of the elderly and aging; type, extent, availability, and accessibility of support; and the level of internal family unit stress. These elements are summarized in Table 1.

Blazer (1982) also points out that frequent, good quality interaction among family members is a positive characteristic for the older

TABLE 1

ELEMENTS OF FAMILY EVALUATION FOR THE FAMILY OF THE OLDER ADULT

Family members and family structure

Definition of the family
Individual characteristics of
  family members
Physical location of family members
Roles and role relationsips

Family interaction

Frequency of family interaction
Quality of family interaction
  Compatible versus conflictual
  Cohesive versus fragmented
  Productive versus nonproductive
  Fragile versus stable
  Rigid versus flexible

Family atmosphere

Tensive versus related
Hopeful versus resigned

Family values

Values concerning health and health
Values concerning the elderly

Family support and tolerance

Availability
Tangible supportive services, i.e.,
  generic services
Perception of intangible support
  Dependability
  Interaction
  Belongingness
  Intimacy
  Usefulness
Family tolerance of disturbing
  behaviors

Family stress

From D. Blazer, Depression in Late Life. St. Louis, C.V. Mosby, 1982, p. 223.

depressed member. Similarly, a family which values older members as useful and productive and includes them in family activities, discussions, and decisions offers a more positive environment than a family system which devalues age and perceives older members as a useless burden and bother. Blazer (1980) identified four "intangible supports" which are particularly important for the depressed family member: a dependable social network, social participation or interaction; belongingness and intimacy.

Blazer (1982) offers several suggestions to those treating the family of a depressed older adult. First, he recommends the family be taught the nature of depression in late life and the risk of suicide, as well as how to read the warning signs and clues to depression and suicide. He suggests that the practitioner should carefully explain the nature of the illness and assure family members that comments made by the depressed elder should not be taken personally. The practitioner can instruct family members on how to communicate with the depressed elder and encourage positive interactions. Family members should be encouraged to openly express and discuss their feelings.

Treatment of depression is a major factor in suicide prevention. The spectrum of agents useful in the treatment of affective illness in the elderly includes: monamine oxidase inhibitors, tricyclic antidepressants, lithium, neuroleptics, sedative-anxiolytics, and central stimulants. Electroconvulsive therapy is also effective. The following therapies have all proven effective in combating depression in the old: reminiscence and life review therapy (Lewis and Butler, 1974; Romaniuk and Romaniuk, 1981), creative arts therapy — whether through art, drama, dance, or music (Bright, 1984; Clark and Osgood, 1985; Lerman, 1984), pet therapy (Cusak and Smith, 1984); psychotherapy and group therapy (Horton and Linden, 1982).

Experts agree that the suicidal elderly must be watched carefully for several months after a suicide attempt or serious threat. The most dangerous time is often when things seem to be going very well and the older individual seems to have "recovered" from his or her depression.

Active outreach and education of service providers, older adults, and the public are also necessary components of any large-scale effort to prevent suicide among older adults.

REFERENCES

Ackerman, N. (1985). *The psychodynamics of family life*. New York: Basic Books.

Bengtson, V. L. & Treas, J. (1980). The changing family context of mental health and aging. In J. E. Birren & R. B. Sloane (Eds.), *Handbook of mental health and aging* (pp. 400-428). Engelwood Cliffs, NJ: Prentice-Hall.

Berardo, F. (1970). Survivorship and social isolation: The case of the aged widower. *Family Coordinator, 19*, 11-25.

Blazer, D. (1980). *Social supports and mortality in a community population*. Ph.D. dissertation, University of North Carolina. Chapel Hill.

Blazer, D. (1982). *Depression in late life*. St. Louis: C. V. Mosby.

Bright, R. (1972). *Music in geriatric care*. New York: St. Martins Press.

Brody, E. H. (1966). The aging family. *Gerontologist, 6*, 201-206.

Brody, E. H. & Spark, G. M. (1966). Institutionalization of the elderly: A family crisis. *Family Process, 5*, 76-90.

Caplan, G. (1976). The family as a support system. In G. Caplan & M. Killilea (Eds.), *Support systems and mutual help: Multidisciplinary explorations* (pp. 19-36). New York: Grune and Stratton.

Cath, S. H. (1965). Discussion notes. In M. A. Berezin & S. H. Cath (Eds.), *Geriatric psychiatry: Grief, loss, and emotional disorders of the aging process*. New York: International University Press.

Clark, P. & Osgood, N. J. (1985). *Seniors on stage: The impact of applied theatre techniques on the elderly*. New York: Praeger.

Cuszak, O. & Smith, E. (1984). *Pets and the elderly: The therapeutic bond*. New York: The Haworth Press, Inc.

Durkheim, E. (1951). *Suicide: A study in sociology*. New York: Free Press.

Farberow, N. L. & Shneidman, E. S. (1970). Suicide and age. In E. S. Shneidman, N. L. Farberow, & R. E. Litman (Eds.), *The psychology of suicide*. New York: Science House.

Freud, S. (1917). *Mourning and melancholia*. Collected papers IV. repr. Hogarth Press, London, 1948.

Gottesman, I. E., Quarterman, C. E. & Cohn, G. M. (1973). Psychosocial treatment of the aged. In C. Eisdorfer & M. P. Lawton (Eds.), *Psychology of adult development and aging*. Washington, DC: American Psychological Association.

Gubrium, J. (1974). Marital desolation and the evaluation of everyday life in old age. *Journal of Marriage and the Family, 36*, 107-113.

Gurland, B. J. & Cross, P. S. (1983). Suicide among the elderly. In M. K. Aronson, R. Bennett, & B. T. Gurland (Eds.), *The acting out elderly* (pp. 456-65). New York: The Haworth Press, Inc.

Herr, J. J. & Weakland, J. H. (1979). *Counseling elders and their families: Practical techniques for applied gerontology*. New York: Springer.

Horton, A. M. & Linden, M. E. (1982). Geriatric group psychotherapy. In A. Horton (Ed.), *Mental health intervention for the aging* (pp. 52-68). New York: Praeger Press.

Kastenbaum, R. (1985, July). *"Why go on?" Suicidal thoughts and actions in later life*. Paper presented at the 13th Meeting of the International Congress on Gerontology, New York.

Lerman, L. (1984). *Teaching dance to senior adults*. Springfield, IL: Thomas.

Lewis, M. L. & Butler, R. N. (1974). Life-review therapy: Putting memories to work in individual and group psychotherapy. *Geriatrics, 29* (1), 165-173.

Madanes, C. (1981). *Strategic family therapy*. San Francisco: Jossey Bass.

McIntosh, J. L. (1985). *Suicide among minority elderly*. Paper presented at the Annual Meeting of the Gerontological Society of America.

McIntosh, J. L. (1984). Components of the decline in elderly suicide: Suicide among the young-old and old-old by race and sex. *Death Education, 8* (Supplement), 113-124.

McIntosh, J. L. & Santos, J. F. (1981). Suicide among minority elderly: A preliminary investigation. *Suicide and Life-Threatening Behavior, 11*, 151-166.

Menninger, K. (1938). *Man against himself*. New York: Harcourt, Brace & World.

Miller, M. (1979). *Suicide after sixty: The final alternative*. New York: Springer.

Murray, R., Huelskoetter, M. & O'Driscoll, D. (1980). *The nursing process in later maturity*. Englewood Cliffs, NJ: Prentice-Hall.

National Center for Health Statistics (1985). Advance report of final mortality statistics 1983 *NCHS Monthly Vital Statistics Report* 34 (6, Supplement 2).

Richman, J. (1986). *Family therapy for suicidal people*. New York: Springer.

Romaniuk, M. & Romaniuk, J. (1981). Looking back: An analysis of reminiscence functions and triggers. *Experimental Aging Research, 7*(4), 477-489.

Rosow, I. (1967). *Social integration of the aged*. New York: Free Press.

Sainsbury, P. (1963). Social and epidemiological aspects of suicide with special reference to the aged. In R. H. Williams, C. Tibbitts & W. Donahue (Eds.), *Processes of aging: Social and psychological perspectives* (Vol. 2, pp. 151-176). New York: Atherton.

Savitsky, E. & Sharkey, I. (1972). The geriatric patient and his family: Study of family interaction in the aged. *Journal of Geriatric Psychiatry, 5* (1), 3-24.

Seiden, R. (1981). Mellowing with age: Factors influencing the nonwhite suicide rate. *International Journal of Aging and Human Development, 13* (4), 265-281.

Shanas, E. & Streib, G. (Eds.) (1965). *Social structure and the family: Generational relations*. Englewood Cliffs, NJ: Prentice-Hall.

Weiss, R. S. (1976). Transition states and other stressful situations: Their nature and programs for their management. In G. Caplan & M. Killilea (Eds.), *Support systems and mutual help: Multidisciplinary explorations* (pp. 213-222). New York: Grune & Stratton.

Roles of the Psychotherapist in Family Financial Counseling: A Systems Approach to Prolongation of Independence

Richard L. D. Morse

SUMMARY. A systems approach is provided the psychotherapist, beginning with the development of factual profiles: of client's income, expenses, and net worth, and of the client's social network, identifying right to and claims on other persons and institutions. In the process of developing the data based profiles, there will arise opportunity to evaluate the adequacy of the current status and provisions made for the future. The need for consumer alertness is emphasized, as is having a proper respect for the limitations of money. The paper closes with a series of questions appropriate for all ages, but especially the older persons whose "count down" years become increasingly finite.

The working premise of this paper is that the foundation of "good" old age, that which prolongs independent living, rests on three supports: good health, good feeling of self-worth and good sense of economic security. While the focus of this paper is on money and economic security, it is not to the exclusion of the other two elements. To do otherwise would be to reduce the discussion to the mathematics of finance and standard professional approaches to personal finance and consumer protection.

All three are interrelated and should be considered in working with clients. The interrelationship may be illustrated by a person in need of money to buy dentures. But money alone might not be the

---

Richard L. D. Morse, PhD, is Professor of Family Economics, Kansas State University, Manhattan, KS 66502.

133

answer. It could be used to buy lottery tickets rather than teeth. It could buy poor (unacceptable) teeth or teeth that fit perfectly, depending on availability and exercise of good buymanship skill in the selection of professional services. The money, translated into functional dentures, would thereby allow buying foods formerly too difficult to chew, and this could lead to better nutrition, more energy and better health, or, to increased volume of junk foods with high cholesterol, fat and salt. So, if money and health are interrelated, how about self-worth? In terms of mental attitude, every bite with the newly purchased teeth may bring a reminder of the humbling experience of accepting money from a charity agency, a well-meaning son-in-law or public welfare; it could bring back feelings of disappointment with health insurance coverage and the niggardliness of government programs that do not pay for dentures, or the "overcharges" of the dentist. On the other hand, the money spent for these teeth could bring joy of seeing one's picture with a full smile instead of an embarrassed clenched jaw occasioned by the photographer's plea: "Now let's all smile." Money, therefore, can lead to wasteful spending, or it can contribute to an improved quality of life.

The ultimate effect on a person's quality of life depends on balancing: (1) scientific facts about what is or is not possible, with (2) application of these facts to the social and market situation—product and service availability, transportation, sales promotion and resistance, with (3) ability to assess and understand individual needs, together with willingness to experiment with something new and different, and to take risks, and with (4) the ability to integrate these strands of influence into a decision-making mode that is comfortable to the clients, advances their health and sense of well being, and is within budget. The integration of the fruits of such knowledge and its application to specific situations, however, presents a responsible role for family therapists to whom this paper is addressed.

It is the purpose of this paper to provide the psychotherapist with a realistic approach to financial counseling that will assist them in helping clients prolong independence.

UNDERSTANDING THE ROLE OF MONEY

Money is not only a means to good health and feeling of self-worth, but also to a feeling of economic security and of economic adequacy. However, this should not be confused with freedom from economic pressure.

Economic pressure is normal and even desirable. This is a useful statement, for it underscores the fact that economic pressure is not directly a function of the amount of money. For example, low-income families, people from remotely rural areas, and many elderly may feel under less economic pressure than the upward mobile, aspiring "yuppie" junior executive who anticipates next year's raise to cover last year's credit balances.

Economic pressure is a function of the distance between level of income and what it buys and the cost of the living desired. Some persons need to have their aspirations raised while others need to restore realism to their expectations, keeping them within their means. This is always a delicate balance, requiring an art of living rather than compliance with a "scientific"-objective-average-budget prepared by experts. Some persons are better than others in coping with this challenge. Others may experience difficulty as they move into new life styles as a result of life-cycle changes. The elderly in retirement may need the help of the psychotherapist in understanding and adjusting to major shifts in the economic equations of life: For example, they often must adjust from thinking in terms of wages and salary that increase with the cost of living and that reward their productivity into thinking in terms of a future of relatively static money income from social security, pensions, annuities, IRA payouts, etc. Their plight is further confounded upon observing their young replacement back at the old job getting higher and higher salaries. Indeed, they must behave more cautiously. Spirited risk taking is for the younger who have recovery time from losses that is not available to the older person whose time is running out. They may need help adjusting to surges in income and expenses, such experienced by the widow who may receive a windfall from an estate, or be devastated by not only her husband's death, but the final medical bills.

For the first time in life, the older person must begin to think in terms of "count down" years and to learn first hand from peers of the inadequacy of medical care insurance coverage and how costs have forced them to be dependent upon family, friends, or welfare. They have good reason to be haunted by the specter of long term nursing home costs eroding savings, leaving the surviving spouse destitute.

The family therapist can help clients work through most of the unanswerable questions that grow out of this maneuvering between what one has and what one wants in such a manner that individual self-esteem is enhanced, and thereby retain a feeling of being in command of their own situation. The systems approach suggested for use by the psychotherapist in dealing with the client is to: (1) Assess the known facts, (2) Explore alternatives, and (3) Project into the future. Limitations of space will permit only a few suggestions:

1. *The Facts*. (a) Start with last year's income tax returns and trace the sources of income to obtain a realistic picture of what was available to the client. Then work with the client reconstructing the expenditure/savings side to learn where the money went. This paints a picture of the client's "quality of life" as played out by the client. (Incidentally, as you go through this exercise with the client and experience problems of memory recall, you may start thinking of ways to help the client grow in confidence and understanding about the money process by considering making wise use of credit card billing systems, personal allowances, special savings accounts, etc.) Needless to say, there are countless accounting/bookkeeping systems available for organizing such data.

(b) Establish the economic status of the client by drawing up a statement of net worth as of that date, as of the end of the last quarter, or as of some other specific date. This very simple statement can reveal a wealth of baseline information for analysis and evaluation. There are three steps: First, list what they own (certificate #, plat and lot #, bond #, etc.), its market value, who owns it (him, her, joint, children), and where the papers are kept (safe deposit, desk drawer, etc.) and recorded. Next, list what is owed, how much, and to whom. Here again be specific. Finally, compute the difference to determine what they are worth, NET. One dramatic approach is to assume momentary death and view the process of valuing an estate that would be distributed under state law or by will. That is a simple and crisp scenario. But since your client plans on living, this net worth statement can provide a realistic data base for your client to think about what needs, hopes and aspirations that sum might provide. Indeed, you may expect two reactions from the client: Initially, it might be, "Didn't know we had so much!" and followed later by: "Why that won't go as far as I had hoped it would." (See step 3.)

(c) Establish a profile of the support/responsibility pattern of this client for four levels: (i) Within the immediate family/household; who can be expected to do what for whom. (ii) Within the extended family, from whom can support be expected, and to what extent does the client feel a sense of obligation to help others? Economic pressures vary considerably with the number of children and grandparents to support, and, conversely, the children and relatives on whom one can rely. (iii) Outside the family, what support may come from friends, neighbors, church members and organizations within the community, and, in turn, which ones does the client feel required to support. Church members with a "helping hand" attitude offer immeasurably more support than thousands of dollars could buy. (iv) In the larger environment of state, national and international arena in which this client-citizen participates, what support systems may the client rely upon and expect as a right, and, in turn, what obligations does the client feel required to support? A civilized society is one that is organized to contribute care to the needy and demand support from the able, and does so through systems of taxation and distribution or by voluntary contributions and relief. It too often is misunderstood and unappreciated because both the giving and receiving aspects are not properly perceived, especially from the perspective of a potential dependent.

Special attention to this profile is pertinent to the elderly as they experience irreversible revolutions in their life patterns and social-dependency relationships. Not only do family roles change dramatically from rightful independence, if not dominance and respect, to recognition of ultimate dependency. Also, friends, neighbors and service providers also grow older, some becoming less accountable and useful while others become more reliable. The importance of exercising social skills to develop new relationships to replace the old becomes evident. And as society ages, personal adjustments are required to take advantage of services which have developed with the new awareness, such as the nutrition sites and community senior service centers. Programs which might be construed as designed for "those old people" may prove to be quite valuable with changing the pronouns from "those" to "our." If the family therapist can help make this transformation in attitude, the quality of life of clients can be well increased at no money cost.

The Older Americans Act has provided networks to assist older citizens enjoy a better quality of life in senior centers and community nutrition sites. The provision of low income and moderate income housing has made living in decent housing affordable. On the other hand, medical economics, cost and cheap cures, frighten many elderly into falling prey to quackery and health insurance fraud schemes. And the billings following an episode of illness from hospitals, doctors, clinics, Blue Cross/Shield, Medicare bewilder the elderly and even cause many younger persons to question their own ability to comprehend. Families living in countries with national health plans providing for those in need regardless of economic status are "richer" than families living in countries with high cost billing and reimbursement systems that are so confusing and offer no assurance of what future costs will be.

Standardized forms for organizing and recording such important information are not available. But the mere process of developing a format and recording such information can be therapeutic. It will draw upon the creative talents of both counselor and client to think through (and to develop an appreciation for) all the potential resources. These nonmarket services often are of the type that make poor people rich, and without which, rich people can be impoverished.

2. *Alternatives to be explored* will emerge in the process of developing the facts profiles. Only a few of the points that may emerge will be cited to illustrate the benefits from this exercise:

+ The income profile will open up questions about alternative sources of income. Some may be tempted to consider work-at-home schemes that too often are fraudulent. The middle class elderly may be surprised to find themselves in the 42% and possibly in the

52.5% marginal income tax bracket and wish to rethink whether they are working for money or for the pleasure of it. (Actually, they may revise their concept of retirement as being relief from "having" to work to working at what they want to do.) Many elderly do learn the difference between working for pay and working for satisfaction. For example, many engage in volunteer activities, such as delivering meals or working in churches because of the satisfaction gained from being needed and being of help, and because of the recreational and social experiences.

+ The net worth statement may stimulate questions about —

— the income it can provide; amount and for how long.

— a host of management questions, particularly if there is a sizable net worth involving property, equities, mutual funds, bonds and CDs.

— the competency of the money manager and his/her proxy or co-manager, and whether a professional trust officer should be engaged.

— pensions, IRAs and other devises that formerly did not seem worthy of serious study, but suddenly are of vital importance to the future.

— about wills, trusts, gifts and ownership; about the use of an *inter vivos* trust to avoid probate to give direction as to disposition of the estate and provide for continuity.

Most of these questions require the services of specialized professionals, the selection of which is a critical and often traumatic experience. Also, it is too often avoided out of fear of being intimidated or overcharged. One of the most helpful roles of the therapist is to assist the client in making such selections as a tax accountant, lawyer, estate planner so the client feels confidently staffed. But more important, the client often needs help in thinking through what work product is expected of each, that is, help in formulating the right questions and deciding which ones require the technical skills of a professional. By this process the client can enter into contracts with professionals with an understanding that may relieve the client later from needless resentment over "excessive" fees for "unnecessary" work. Indeed, the client may come to realize how costly it is to pay others to do what they could do for themselves. They may also realize that the professional will and should not answer for them those tough questions they too often wish to avoid, such as, "What do I want from the remainder of my life?"

+ The rights/responsibility profile has the potential for helping the client relate to others realistically. Indeed it may have the beneficial effect of helping them appreciate the number of unused services their tax dollar provides; they may consider using services of the local library, the school system, the Co-operative Extension Service, the recreation department as well as the senior center and programs of the Area Agency on Aging. And if some of these do not exist or are inadequate, they may explore whether their citizen input might be constructive and how they can contribute to remedy the deficiency. They may find that they are needed and can contribute to the well being of others less fortunate. They may experience the riches that come from sharing. This approach may not be considered financial counseling, yet it can offer richer rewards than money can buy.

3. *Future Projections.* Those who lived through double digit inflation and witnessed their meager savings erode in value, those who cannot adjust to paying one dollar for a ten-cent loaf of bread, or believe a house call from a plumber can be $25 minimum, are fully aware of the futility of projecting economic facts. Yet a better understanding of the extreme parameters may be helpful in distinguishing the probable from the impossible.

In 1975 this author considered his own predictions ridiculous when he said then the ". . . budget level for an elderly couple of $6000 would require $10,916 in 1985 if prices increased at 6%; and $19,802 if the rate of inflation is 12%." By hindsight, this was not far from the truth. Of course, this projection was based on the working of compound interest and can be approximated by applying the "Rule of 72" which is: the number of years required for doubling is 72 divided by an assumed rate. So what costs $10 now will cost $20 in 6 years at a 12% rate, or in 12 years at a 6% rate. Likewise, $10000 invested in a CD at 8% compounded annually will be worth $20000 in 9 years. This simple magic enriches investment counselors who convey a sense of special talent when it is merely the magic of compound interest (Morse, 1975).

The most reliable income source is social security, and its contribution to future security is readily available from the SSA for the asking. Benefits are indexed for inflation, so can be related directly to current living costs to project adequacy for covering the basics of food, clothing, and other routine expenditures. The big unknown is future health care costs, and in considering retirement housing, the provision of long term care should be a high priority. But even the best of plans are only as secure as the financial stability of the institution, for which there is no guarantee. As mentioned, the unknown cost of meeting this final phase of life haunts many elderly. The fear of dying destitute causes many to live in self-denial, holding back on spending for pleasures and even necessities. This is a major social problem that lies outside the scope of this paper.

A big unknown for those contemplating retirement is pension benefits. A recent report of the U.S. Government Accounting Office was issued at Hearings before the Select Committee on Aging of the House of Representatives (Roybal, 1987). It reports that many workers do not know when they can retire. It is equally true that most do not know what those benefits will be. However, the client should be prompted to read the retirement benefit program provisions of employment. This will lead into pertinent personal questions about joint survivorship and guarantee years and their impact on the level of benefits. This is an area in which the client will need help.

This is admittedly extremely limited coverage of this important area of concern and opportunity for client assistance. But it will suffice to indicate the types of matters that require consideration.

CONSUMER ALERTNESS

The true worth of money lies in what it will buy and how it is spent. Excessive use of vitamins even at bargain prices is wasteful. Doctors' prescriptions filled by higher-priced druggists may be convenient, but expensive, especially if filled by brand names rather than generics. Shopping smarts can greatly reduce the cost of living.

Cost of living is determined by what is bought and the prices paid. Shopping around and watching sales, however, may be a privileged activity no longer available to the elderly. Nevertheless, the advent of mail order drugs from the American Association of Retired Persons Pharmacy, for example, could be considered. For example, the annual savings on a cholesterol reducing prescription drug was recently determined to be $205 — a 25% difference. There may be comparable situations which can be explored locally.

The major cost determinant, however, is in the choices made. Choices based on faulty knowledge or misconceptions can be expensive both in term of disappointment, but in displacing a worthy product or service. There may be little role for the psychotherapist other than to encourage reading of *Consumer Reports* and selections from Consumer Union's excellent book list, and using pertinent publications of the Consumer Affairs Division of AARP.

Fraud, quackery and deception are commonly perpetrated on the elderly whose vulnerability is well identified by hucksters and the very sophisticated marketers with their boiler room operations and incessant mailings. Waddell (1975) attributes the susceptibility of older persons to their feelings of loneliness and isolation, experience of grief, desire for restoration of health and vigor, and avoidance of pain and suffering, lower formal education and tendency to be ill-informed, loss of trusted sources of information and their low income level causing them to grasp for income opportunities.

Morse (1980, 1981) emphasizes the unique aspects of older persons that contribute to their unusual consumer problems: changes in life role emphases, economic situations, living arrangements, physiological changes, and shifts in right/responsibility patterns. New consumer coping skills are required with the "new and different" products and services. For example, in only one issue of the *Washington Post* there appeared advertisements of 73 different rates on savings, with continuous, monthly, quarterly, and annual compounding on 365/365 and 365/360 day bases which are a far cry from the 4% quarterly compounded passbook savings accounts of former years (Edwards, 1985). Some of these problems cannot be addressed effectively by the psychotherapist, but by a change in the social-political-economic system, such as adopting a standard interest rate format like Cents-ible Interest® (Morse, 1987) and instituting small claims courts, requiring informative labeling and larger size print, and many other reforms suggested by the Kansas Citizens Council on Aging and embraced at the 1971 White Council on Aging in its session on "The Elderly Consumer" (1971).

The Special Committee on Aging, U.S. Senate, has held hearings and undertaken extensive investigations of frauds and deception affecting the elderly with special attention given to pacemakers, hearing aids, clinical laboratories, vision impairment, elder abuse, unnecessary surgery, medical devices. An informative 18-page booklet, prepared by committee staff, identifies the 10 most harmful frauds and tells how to combat them. It is available from the committee (Senate, 1983). The Select Committee on Aging of the House of Representatives, has done similar productive work and reports are available from that committee.

The family therapist should become familiar with the many sources of assistance, beginning with such local resources as the Area Agency on Aging, the city/county consumer protection agency and the services of the state office of attorney general. At the national level many non-profit agencies publish excellent materials, such as those of the Arthritis Foundation, American Cancer Society, American Heart Association and the Better Business Bureau. And despite the recent trend to deregulate, there remains the Food and Drug Administration (which also includes coverage of medical devices and cosmetics), the Federal Trade Commission (advertising and marketing), the indomitable U.S. Postal Service (for misuse of mails for health restorers, arthritis cures, worthless medical devices, work-at-home schemes). Religious and charitable organizations too often are flagrant purveyors of fraud and chicanery promising hope of eternal blessedness in return for material contributions. Even though the cause for which money is solicited may be worthy, the portion of the contribution that goes to the charity may be less than that pocketed by the solicitor. Some pleas are so ridiculous one wonders whether there are enough suckers to warrant the effort, such as the one-inch piece of a shirt tail sent a 100-year-old woman with instructions to hold the prayer cloth and pray to God for a special miracle and a divine touch for a special friend, to write down those requests and insert them along with a contribution in an envelope for mailing back to the Rev. Blank Blank of Phoenix. He would pray for 3 days and 3 nights with the prayer cloth and then return it to be carried "as a sign of our united faith for your SPECIAL MIRACLE." The request is rationalized by this quote from an insert: "God often uses foolish things to confound the wise (1 Corinthians 1:27)."

THE COUNTDOWN

The inevitability of death becomes increasingly real with aging, and it is often accompanied by anxiety about how many of the questions that surround the event of death will be answered. These unanswered questions can plague the living. The questions may range from profound concerns for the care of the surviving spouse to a somewhat trivial matter as to who will get the teapot or be among the pallbearers. Some of these questions may be so difficult the client prefers to let them be answered by default. Many can be answered with the stimulation of an interested outside person providing guidance and assurance, and willingness to put the wishes into a formal written document. In many situations, the client may not have a clear understanding of what death involves and would welcome having the full slate of questions presented so they can be addressed and dispensed with. Actually, the process of raising questions may lead to further questions. But it can be anticipated that in running through the questions, there will be some that can be readily answered, others that can await further consideration, and those that will require professional technical information. As a result, the client should have a more legitimate feeling of confidence in having made decisions about the most personal aspect of the client's life.

The CHECK LIST proposed is merely to suggest the major points the psychotherapist should cover and would be expected to embellish upon in accordance with his/her professional style and the nature of the client's circumstances.

1. *Have you made funeral plans?*

If yes, what are they? (Are they complete? If there is a prepaid plan, how reliable is it and what flexibility is allowed? Does it include answers to all the questions the funeral director will ask?)

If no, why not? (Follow-up questions would cover cost estimates and provision for payment; method of disposing of the body, including donation of organs; form of ceremony desired; who should make the decisions, and all the other details concerned with making funeral arrangements.)

2. *Do you have any heirs or dependents?* (See the rights/responsibility profile.)

3. *How long do you expect to live*, and for your spouse and other dependents to live? What is your and their health status, family history of health problems, and prediction of need for long term care? (The IRA tables of estimated life would be a useful guide.)

4. *Have you made a will?*

If yes, where is it? When was it last reviewed? Does it still reflect your wishes? Would you be unhappy if following your death there was a family settlement agreement by which the family changed the disposition of your estate? Do you object to having your estate made a matter of public record?

If no, why not? Did you neglect it? Do you not care and prefer to have the survivors "fight it out" or develop their own settlement agreement? Or, do you feel the state law provides for an equitable distribution? Or have you placed all real property into joint ownership with right of survivorship so it will pass automatically? And, have you listed your personal property and noted to whom it should go at death? Or have you placed your holdings into an *inter vivos* trust, making yourself a trustee with your survivor as contingent trustee to take over upon your death?

5. *Have you drawn up a statement of net worth* as described in the preceding? Have you reviewed this with the thought of how the "surplus" should be used, or for how the "deficit" and debts should be handled? Do you have in mind "living up" your estate? Or do you wish to continue to live as now, and to leave the residue to charity, your children and grandchildren?

6. *What would you like to do in the next five years?* What would this involve? What are the major obstacles to your achieving this?

7. Repeat this question *for additional time segments* to pace the life expectations with abilities in declining years.

This line of questions can be expected to raise a host of questions that may demand attention of those trained in tax accounting, probate law, estate planning. But the role of the psychotherapist is to assist the client in framing the appropriate questions, to help the client negotiate with outside professionals and contract for only those services needed, not allowing the professional to enlarge on the scope of work and cost (as is often their inclination), and then to help the client put the pieces of information into a whole with which the client feels comfortable and can go about enjoying life.

CONCLUSION

In summary the role of the psychotherapist is to assist the client to integrate the essentials of good health, good feeling of self-worth and good sense of economic security in such manner as to enhance those feelings of independence that are essential for better living. The approach suggested is to start with the factual data to be developed with the client to reveal the economic status of the client and profile the client's life style in relation to other persons and use of money. Out of the process of data collection will emerge a host of questions that will prompt further questions with which the client can be assisted. The special position of the older person as consumer is acknowledged. A series of "count down" questions is suggested because these are universally applicable to all, but moreso for the older person.

REFERENCES

Edwards, Donna O. (1985). *Elderly's perception of interest rate quotations on savings*. Unpublished master's thesis. Kansas State University, Manhattan.

Morse, Richard L. D. (1975). Could the marketplace be more responsive to the needs of older consumers? In *Proceedings, National Forum on Consumer Concerns of Older Americans*, American Association of Retired Persons: Washington, DC., pp. 52-61.

Morse, Richard L. D. (1980). Consumers all. In *Handbook on Aging*. American Home Economics Association: Washington, DC.

Morse, Richard L. D. (1981). The economics of aging. *Hort Therapy*, 1(2):13-18. National Council for Therapy and Rehabilitation Through Horticulture: Alexandria, VA.

Morse, Richard L. D. (1987). Truth in savings — its legislative history and status. In *Proceedings, 33rd Annual Conference*, American Council on Consumer Interests: Columbia, MO. pp. 51-57.

Roybal, Edward R. (1987). Workers don't know when to retire. *Hearing, Select Committee on Aging*, U.S. House of Representatives, September 23, 1987, Washington, DC.

U.S. Senate. (1983). *Consumer frauds and elderly persons: a growing problem.*

An information paper prepared by the staff of the Special Committee on Aging: Washington, DC.

Waddell, Frederick E. (1975). Consumer research and programs for the elderly — the forgotten dimension. *The Journal of Consumer Affairs*, 9(2);164-175.

White House Conference on Aging. (1971). *Report Volume II*. Superintendent of Documents, Washington, DC, pp. 17-23.

Sexual Dysfunction in the Elderly: Causes and Effects

James E. Garrison, Jr.

SUMMARY. This paper examines the fact that sexual expression among the elderly is normal. It also explores the fact that sexual dysfunctions which arise for this age group are basically very similar to those of other age groups, except for those which are organic in nature resulting from the normal aging process. The role of medication and health issues as they relate to sexual dysfunction are discussed as well as the psychological and relationship problems which contribute to dysfunction. In discussing treatment options, special attention is given to issues such as history taking, information sharing, being single, and therapy approaches.

INTRODUCTION

In our culture there is a stereotype that sex and the older generation just do not go together (Kaas & Rousseau, 1983; Comfort, 1980). It is true that the frequency of intercourse and/or orgasms do decline as one ages but a lessening of frequency does not mean that the older generation is asexual. With a sexually interested and interesting partner and with relatively good health one may maintain sexual activity well into his/her eighties and beyond. This does not mean that one has to be sexually active. Rather, it is the good news that one can be sexually active (Thomas, 1982; Weg, 1983).

We know that men have more organically based sexual dysfunctions in the sixty-plus age group than women in that same age group. The main dysfunction for men is impotence, while dyspa-

James E. Garrison, Jr., received his PhD from Virginia Polytechnic Institute and State University and is a licensed professional counselor in private practice of marriage and family therapy at 2727 South Main St., Blacksburg, VA 24060.

reunia (painful intercourse) appears to be one of the main ones for women. Both of these can also have nonorganic causes and the choice of treatment modality must take this into consideration. In addition to the previously mentioned, the obvious dysfunction that is shared by both sexes is the apparent loss of desire to have any sexual relationship at all.

Out of a lack of information about and understanding of the normal physiological changes that accompany aging, many couples withdraw from any chance of sexual fulfillment long before physically required to do so. Societal expectations for the elderly may also cause them to refrain from any sexual experience. Or, physical illness may require the couple to adapt their way of approaching each other sexually. It is important that information about and understanding of the normal sexual development as one ages be shared with the elderly and others who deal with them. Men and women are affected sexually in different ways as they age.

PHYSICAL FACTORS

Changes in Males

Knowledge of the normal physiosexual changes in the male may be helpful to both the man who has a concern about his sexual functioning and his partner. The research of Masters and Johnson (1966, 1970) has demonstrated that there is a decreased production of testosterone until it stabilizes around the age of 60. This decrease may cause a reduction in size and firmness of the testicles. There is reduced sperm production and therefore a lesser chance of impregnation.

Other noticeable changes pointed out are due to changes in the prostate gland. It increases in size with age, especially after the age of 40. Prostatitis, or inflammation of the prostate, is relatively common. The symptoms include pain in the pelvic area, backache, urinary complications including a decrease in urine flow, and maybe a cloudy discharge from the penis. Usually it is treated with antibiotics and massage of the gland. However, if tumors are present treatment may include removal of part or all of the gland. Absence of hormones from the prostate can lead to a lack of erection. In addition the sphincter valves can be damaged by the partial surgery which might result in retrograde ejaculation. With radical surgery, the loss of erectile ability may occur. However, new surgical procedures hold hope for eliminating the threat of this side effect (Glasgow, Halfin, & Althausen, 1987).

A number of changes occur in the sexual response cycle as the male ages. According to Masters and Johnson (1981) these changes begin with a delay in the erection response during the excitement phase. As the man ages more direct stimulation of the penis may be required for an erection and the erection may not be as full or rigid as it was when he was younger. In the plateau phase, the pre-ejaculatory state can be maintained for a much longer period of time. This can be an asset to the sexual relationship since the female receives more stimulation and might reach an orgasm more easily. The orgasm phase for the man is of much shorter duration. There is a reduced sense of urgency and inevitability to ejaculate and there is a diminished volume of seminal fluid accompanied by reduced expulsive force in the ejaculation. The resolution phase is characterized by a shorter time period from orgasm to penile flacidity. A longer refractory period is obvious and often requires from 12 to 24 hours or longer before another erection can occur. This is often lengthened by anxiety over the rapid detumescence and fear that another erection will not occur. The period of time between erections and orgasms increases as the man ages.

Some writers support the theory that the more active a man is sexually in his youth and middle age, the more active he can remain in his later years (Pfeiffer, 1978). Kaplan (1974) points out that if the male and his partner are able to adapt and utilize special techniques which rely heavily on direct physical stimulation of genitals and other erogenous areas he will have a very good chance to remain sexually active into advanced years. If, however, the man ceases to have sex during his 50s and 60s as a result of avoiding the painful realization that he is no longer able to perform as he did in his youth, then impotence will most likely result with varying degrees of permanence. The major stated reason for decrease in sexual activity for men is impotence (Baikie, 1984). However, with the reduction of pressure for rapid orgastic release and the loss of inhibitions of earlier years, the man is often able to enjoy a much more satisfying sexual relationship with his partner (Kaplan, 1974).

Changes in Females

Even though the obvious changes in sexual functioning are not as great as with men, there are changes in the female (Masters & Johnson, 1966, 1970). After the age of 45-50, menopause will occur. Ovarian estrogen slows down (if the ovaries are still present). With the altered ratio of hormones, and the fear of pregnancy being removed, there will often be an increase in sexual desire. (With some women, however, sexual desire decreases since there is no longer a "purpose" in having sex.) Hot flashes occur as a result of hormonal imbalances. Vaginal mucosa becomes thinner and changes to a lighter pinkish color. The length and width of the vagina decrease and there is a diminished expansive ability of the inner vagina during sexual arousal. There is also a reduction of lubrication during sexual response which can result in more painful intercourse.

These changes result in alterations in the response cycle for women in later years. In the excitement phase, lubrication begins more slowly and there is less volume. The sexual flush and expansion of the vagina is less pronounced as one ages but clitoral sensitivity and nipple erection remain. In the plateau phase there is a less dramatic change in the orgasmic platform and uterine elevation. However, the vaginal opening is constricted and the clitoris withdraws under its hood as it would in a younger woman. In the orgasm phase, the number of contractions are reduced and may be experienced as painful by some women. This may be the result of hormone deficiency or imbalance which can be treated by hormone therapy. The resolution after orgasm occurs much more rapidly in post-menopausal women but the woman is fully capable of multiple orgasms, just as when younger (Masters & Johnson, 1981).

Vaginismus, the involuntary constriction of the outer part of the vagina preventing penetration of the penis, may in fact be the result of dyspareunia, painful intercourse which could result from the reduction of lubrication and the loss of elasticity of the vagina itself (Masters & Johnson, 1981).

Many women cease to have intercourse during their 50s and 60s. This abstinence is not necessarily due to the physiological changes already listed. It may be due to psychological and social factors which place the woman as being the more passive partner sexually.

Couples need to be informed of the normal age-related sexual changes which exist. Also they need to be encouraged to adapt to those changes. Brecher (1984) gives excellent examples of how adaptation has been made by aging couples. For example, the changes in coital positions to take into account physical needs, mutual masturbation, more direct genital stimulation, use of lubricants, oral stimulation, non-coitus relationships, and the use of psychological stimulation including fantasy sharing.

Effects of Drugs

The effect of many drugs are exaggerated as one ages, and in particular the effect that certain drugs have on one's sexual performance become greater as one ages. This is particularly true for men where the side effect of temporary impotency is concerned (Felstein, 1983).

If alcohol is abused it may physically produce impotency or the reduction of desire. The alcoholic's behavior when intoxicated may also reduce his/her sexual desirability to the partner. Often used to reduce the anxiety related to sexual activity among the young, alcohol is a central nervous system depressant and has the effect of reducing the performance. This is especially true for the elderly.

High blood pressure medicines, especially some of the older medications, may produce temporary impotency. However there are newer drugs that do not have that side effect.

Antihistamines may produce temporary impotency in the male or reduction of vaginal lubrication which can lead to dyspareunia in the female. This is especially true of many of the "over-the-counter" cold medications. There are now medications available which can avoid this side effect.

A number of psychotropic drugs that are prescribed for the elderly can produce sexual dysfunctions as side effects. Phenothiazines (e.g., Thorazine, or Stelazine) may cause temporary impotence in males. Mellaril tends to cause dry ejaculation, i.e., erection and orgasm occur but there is no ejaculation out of the penis. Butyrophenones (e.g., Haldol) may also cause periods of impotence, reduction of libido, or loss of muscle tone necessary for orgasm.

Antidepressant medications can also cause sexual difficulties. The tricyclics and monamine oxidase inhibitors both may cause temporary impotency. Some coronary care medications may cause impotency and/or loss of sexual desire.

Other Health Issues

Felstein (1983) has pointed out additional health problems which can also lead to sexual dysfunction for the aged. For the female, menopause can often bring on the physical problems mentioned earlier. The feeling of not needing to have sexual relations since she no longer can have children can also occur.

A mastectomy can affect a woman's self-image by causing her to see herself as unattractive and nonsexual. Counseling with the woman and her partner prior to and following surgery can be very beneficial for this problem. Sharing information at this point about types of intimacy and ways of continuing to relate sexually can relieve a great deal of anxiety.

An ovariectomy may produce hormonal imbalances and all of the related physical problems mentioned previously. Some women feel that a part of their sexual identity has been removed when they have a total or partial hysterectomy.

For men, illnesses involving the prostate are very alarming in terms of their sexual functioning. Prostate inflammation or cancer and treatment for these may lead to permanent impotency and/or ejaculatory problems. Testicular cancer treatment, especially if the testicle is removed, can result in a loss of feeling like a total man, emasculated, and therefore, he may not be able to function sexually. It can also cause problems due to reduction of testosterone which can lead to reduction of sexual desire.

Several health issues are of concern to both men and women. For example, a heart attack and/or surgery can produce fear that the excitement or orgasm will bring about another attack resulting in death. This could inhibit either the person with the heart condition or the partner from engaging in any type of sexual relationship. However most advice given recommends that the couple refrain from intercourse for six weeks, after which relatively normal sex relations can resume.

Diabetes can produce sexual problems especially for the male. In about 50% of the males who are diabetic impotency occurs due to nerve damage and decreased blood circulation. The major treatment here is penile implants. For the female diabetic there is a decrease in genital sensation and a reduction in the engorgement of the genitals which results in decreased response and pleasure associated with orgasm.

The main problems related to hypertension come from medication effects which result in loss of erection and/or orgasmic dysfunction. Medication changes can often relieve these dysfunctions.

Cancer related surgeries with ostomies can also cause problems in sexual relationships. The self-image, odor, physical difficulty in having intercourse, are all problematic. Again, counseling prior to and following surgery will aid the patient and his/her partner in adjusting to this problem (Glasgow et al., 1987; Sarrel & Sarrel, 1984). The same approach can aid in dealing with patients who have enuretic or encopretic problems. The sense of embarrassment and loss of a sexual self-image and desire should be the main focus.

The victims of strokes often become concerned that they are no longer attractive to their sexual partners. It is necessary to treat sexual complications in the same light as other factors (Marron, K. R., 1982). Brain damage may contribute to the dysfunction depending on the loss of faculties. There may be a loss of mobility or physical sensations, incontinence, effects of medications as well as cognitive losses, all of which may make sexual relations more difficult and/or unappealing.

PSYCHOLOGICAL ASPECTS

In addition to adjustment to the physical problems mentioned several additional psychological factors may contribute to a reduction of sexual activity as one ages (Comfort, 1980; Corby & Solnick, 1980; Sarrel & Sarrel, 1984). Expressed disinterest in sex may be covering for actual feelings of anxiety over fears of loss of attractiveness or the feeling that the partner has no interest in him/her, whatever the reason (Marron, 1982).

Again, sex may never have been very important to the individual and therefore the level of interest is no different than earlier in life. In addition, expressed disinterest may be secondary to a number of emotional illnesses, e.g., depression, or anxiety. Or it may be the result of boredom in a long term relationship. This is especially true if the partners were not open to experimenting or attempting variations in their sexual relationships.

A reduction in expressed desire may also be an expression of anger or hostility toward the partner. Other family issues may be involved in changes in sexual desire, especially at particular developmental stages such as the launching stage where the parents are having to face each other alone, often for the first time. This reduction in desire then continues into later years with the "excuse" of loss of physical ability. Another vulnerable developmental stage is when the man or woman retires and experiences a great sense of loss of meaning in life.

Rigid moral or religious upbringing may contribute to the lack of expressed desire. The embarrassment over discussing any sexual issues with a physician or counselor can leave the person a victim of his/her own ignorance. The past history and lack of ability to communicate about sexual issues may also prevent any alterations in the physical way they relate to each other. For example if there is an extreme prohibition against masturbation then any form of masturbation as a viable alternative to intercourse would be prohibited, even if intercourse is prohibited due to illness.

The attitude of the elderly being asexual appears to be especially true in our attitudes toward older women. Belsky (1984), in summarizing several studies at Duke University, points out that in our culture aging women are not seen as being sexually attractive. They are expected to be asexual at an earlier age than men. Society appears to have given the message to older women that they are not supposed to be sexual. However the greatest deterrent to sexual activity in women still is the lack of availability of a partner (Belsky, 1984).

If the woman interprets her husband's normal decline in sexual activity as a rejection of her then there is a false basis for anger and distancing in the relationship. If the wife also becomes angry at her husband for not being able to have an erection when she wants him to have one, then the likelihood of his having an erection is very remote.

The couple needs to have a higher degree of openness with each other, love and acceptance to bring to a sexual dysfunction in order to enhance their love relationship. The ability to adapt one's techniques as required by the changes brought about by aging comes only out of that sense of openness and sharing. More intensive sexual therapy may be necessary to deal with dysfunctions at this level. The relationship issues need to be discussed in any of the dysfunctions, but especially in the psychologically originated dysfunctions.

MAJOR DYSFUNCTIONS

The major dysfunctions for the older age group include impotence of men, dyspareunia for women and loss of desire for either.

Impotence in Men

We have seen that impotence is a very real problem for the aging man. The majority of cases of impotence are due to psychological problems. Tests can be performed to determine if the man has nocturnal erections. If the man does have erections during the night then the impotence is not caused by some physical or organic problem as described earlier. If the impotence is psychologically caused, it needs to be treated through sex therapy which focuses on both the individual's performance anxiety and the relationship issues.

Masters and Johnson (1970) have prescribed a method called sensate focus as one way to reduce the anxiety and begin to bring the couple closer in their sexual expression. Through the mutual giving and receiving of caresses which takes the focus off of the erection the couple can begin to recognize that erections can occur and the pressure to have intercourse before the erection is lost can then be reduced. The way of relating sexually can then grow to include a variety of means other than only through intercourse and thereby reduce the pressure to relate mainly through an erection. Janson (1981) has even espoused a technique of the male using the flacid penis to caress the woman's clitoris and vulva until the woman has an orgasm. This could take a great deal of pressure off of the male to have to have an erection and thereby may allow an erection to occur spontaneously.

If the impotence is based on some organic problem, for example as a result of diabetes, the male can achieve an erection by means of one of two types of implants. One is through implantation of flexible "rods" into the penis so that the penis remains semi-erect all of the time. The other allows the man to "pump up" an erection when desired by means of a pump, placed in the lower abdomen, which pumps fluid into two cylinders implanted in the penis making it firm enough for insertion into the vagina during intercourse. Once intercourse is over, the fluid in the cylinders is emptied back into a reservoir to await the next time intercourse is desired. The only drawback is the cost and the possibility that the body might not accept the cylinders. Yet these procedures can be of benefit to a great number of men who are experiencing organically induced impotence.

"Stuffing" a flaccid or semierect penis into the vagina will sometimes bring on an erection (Annon, 1976). This occurs as a result of the sensations felt from being in the vagina.

Female Dyspareunia

If dyspareunia results from a hormone imbalance it can be aided through hormone treatment and the use of a lubricant such as K-Y Jelly to replace the lack of lubrication. When it is the result of a psychological issue then it needs to be treated with intensive sex therapy where personal and relationship issues are taken into account.

Loss of Desire

The loss of desire can be based on the relationship of the sexual partners, the societal expectations, or hormonal changes. Relationship and societal issues can best be dealt with through sex therapy.

The loss of desire resulting from hormone imbalances can be treated by hormone therapy.

THERAPY ISSUES

Model for Sex Therapy

Annon (1976) has espoused a sex therapy model which has a great deal of relevance for dealing with the elderly (Kaas & Rousseau, 1983). His PLISSIT model begins with giving permission to the person or couple to be sexual in any way they may desire. This sets the groundwork allowing the clients to talk about sexual issues. The next step moves to providing information to the client or couple where only limited information was present. This is illustrated by the sharing of normal developmental facts in order to alter specific expectations. The third aspect of Annon's model is that of giving specific suggestions. The therapist/physician can provide suggestions which are tailored to the unique needs and personality of the client and his/her partner. The last part of the model which Annon presents is intensive therapy which addresses the deeper relationship issues and barriers an individual may have regarding his/her own sexuality.

History Taking

When a therapist or physician is presented with a sexual dysfunction, it is essential to do a thorough history of the problem in order to determine the best therapeutic approach. It is recommended that the following areas be covered:

— Detail of problem: What, when, where, how the problem (dysfunction) occurs.
— History of past occurrence.
— History of relationship: non-sexual.
— History of relationship: sexual.
— History of family of origin with particular emphasis of the family's attitude and messages about sex and sexuality.
— Occurrence of any stressors both in the individual or the family — both nuclear and extended.

— Medical/health history, with particular attention to medications being taken.
— Expectations of both the person with the dysfunction and his/her partner regarding their sexual relationship.

Societal Attitudes

Attitudes and expectations which society has toward the elderly being sexually active present a number of problems for the elderly. This shows up in the attitudes of the young toward the elderly and in the outcries of many adult children who feel their elderly parents are acting out in some abnormal sexual manner. These attitudes and expectations often make the elderly defensive about their normal sexual desires.

The general belief of the elderly being asexual also may have brought on much premature impotence, guilt, frustration and loneliness in that the elderly may have taken it as the way they are supposed to feel or act. They may have also been facilitated in owning this feeling of guilt by their physician who may not be accepting of the sexual feelings of the elderly.

The aversion of physicians and counselors may be the result of that professional's inability to accept his/her parents' intimate relationships. Thus when one talks to elderly clients it becomes extremely uncomfortable because these are sexual matters in which one's parents may have been involved. This is especially true if the elderly person is unmarried.

It is essential to be aware that with good health, a sense of self-awareness, and communication with their partner the elderly can maintain sexual relationships well into their advanced years. Starr and Weier (1981) have given an excellent guide to the elderly as they attempt to improve their sexual relationships.

Therapist Issues

When one sees an elderly person, in regard to sexual problems, do not presume that person is married. The person may be single and yet have a sexual partner of the opposite or same sex. The same types of problems happen for those outside of marriage as for those in it and a number of elderly have relationships without being married. Homosexual relationships also continue into old age and they often experience the same type of dysfunctions mentioned above which need to be treated with the same techniques.

Education of the elderly person, his/her family members, and institutional staff can aid in recognizing the sexual nature of the elderly. This might also increase the variety of ways they can find closeness and intimacy (Svilard, 1978).

Language may need to be adapted to the client keeping in mind the value system in which the client was raised. He/she may not be used to speaking explicitly about sexual relationships. But it is essential the therapist deal with the issues forthrightly in a spirit of understanding and patience in order to prevent misunderstandings as to the nature of the problem.

CONCLUSION

When one is working with the elderly concerning sexual dysfunctions it is essential that a good history be taken. This can then help determine if the dysfunction is physical in origin or if psychological problems are the cause. This distinction will help determine the modality of treatment. Should the problem be approached through information sharing, permission giving or more involved sex therapy? Should the person be treated alone or with his/her partner? Does the physical aspect of the dysfunction need to be treated through changes in the medication or through surgical procedures.

The therapist or physician must be aware of his/her own feeling about the sexual activity of the elderly and be willing to address sexual issues as he/she would any other issue. Issues regarding sexual fulfillment need to be seen not as essential to health but as enrichment to life.

REFERENCES

Annon, J. S. (1974). *Behavioral treatment of sexual problems: Brief therapy*. Hagerstown, MD: Harper & Row, Publishers.

Baikie, E. (1984). Sexuality and the elderly. In I. Hanley & J. Hodge (Eds.), *Psychological approaches to the care of the elderly*. London: Croom Helm.

Belsky, J. K. (1984). *The psychology of aging: theory, research, and practice*. Monterey, CA: Brooks/Cole Publishing Company.

Brecher, E. M. (1984). *Love, sex and aging*. Boston: Little, Brown & Co.

Comfort, A. (1980). Sexuality in late life. In J. E. Birren & R. B. Sloane, (Eds.), *Handbook of mental health and aging*. Englewood Cliffs, NJ: Prentice-Hall.

Corby, N., & Solnick, R. L. (1980). Psychosocial and Physiological influences on sexuality in the older adult. In J. E. Birren & R. B. Sloane (Eds.), *Handbook of mental health and aging*. Englewood Cliffs, NJ: Prentice-Hall.

Felstein, I. (1983). Dysfunction: Origin and therapeutic approaches. In R. Weg (Ed.), *Sexuality in the later years: Roles and behavior*, (pp. 223-247). New York: Academic Press.

Glasgow, M., Halfin, V., & Althausen, A. F. (1987). Sexual response and cancer. *CA-Cancer Journal For Clinicians, 37*(6), 322-332.

Janson, W. J. (1981). *Sexual pleasure sharing*. Jaffrey, NH: Human Development Publications.

Kaas, M. J., & Rousseau, G. K. (1983). Geriatric sexual conformity: Assessment and intervention. *Clinical Gerontologist, 2*(1), 31-44.

Kaplan, H. S. (1974). *The new sex therapy*. New York: Brunner/Mazel, Publishers.

Marron, K. R. (1982). Sexuality with aging. *Geriatrics, 37*(9), 135-138.

Masters, W. H., & Johnson, V. E. (1966). *Human sexual response*. Boston: Little, Brown and Co.

Masters, W. H., & Johnson, V. E. (1970). *Human sexual inadequacy*. Boston: Little, Brown & Co.

Masters, W. H., & Johnson, V. E. (1981). Sex and the aging process. *Journal of American Geriatric Society, 29*, 385-390.

Pfeiffer, E. (1975). Sexual behavior. In J. G. Howells (Ed.), *Modern perspectives in the psychiatry of old age*, (pp. 313-25). London: Churchill Livingston.

Sarrel, B. D., & Sarrel, P. M. (1984). *Sexual turning points: The seven stages of adult sexuality*. New York: MacMillan Publishing Co.

Starr, B. D., & Weiner, M. B. (1981). *On sex and sexuality in the mature years*. New York: Stein & Day.

Sviland, M. A. P. (1978). Helping elderly couples become sexually liberated: Psychosocial issues. In J. LoPiccolo, & LoPiccolo, L. (Eds.), *Handbook of sex therapy*, (pp. 351-360). New York: Plenum Press.

Thomas, L. E. (1982). Sexuality and aging: Essential vitamin or popcorn? *The Gerontologist, 22*(3), 240-243.

Weg, R. (1983). Introduction: Beyond intercourse and orgasm. In R. Weg (Ed.), *Sexuality in the later years: Roles and behavior*, (pp. 1-10). New York: Academic Press.

Legal Ramifications of Elderly Cohabitation: Necessity for Recognition of Its Implications by Family Psychotherapists

Doryce Sanders Hughston
George A. Hughston

SUMMARY. This paper views cohabitation among the elderly from a legal perspective and presents realities of which many family practitioners may not be aware. Five key areas that the therapist and his or her clients should recognize will provide a foundation for understanding the responsibilities and potential legacy of the cohabitation. By design, this paper should contribute to the avoidance of the costly and unpleasant resort to legal suit. An appended list of 28 legally-oriented items should be considered at the outset of cohabitation.

INTRODUCTION

In one of the more practical descriptions, systems theory has been equated to an automobile. An automobile consists of component parts, linked together, in order to accomplish a specific purpose, that is, moving from Point A to Point B. Each part functions in coordination with other parts and, by design, is necessary for the effective and smooth operation of the vehicle. Should problems

Doryce Sanders Hughston is affiliated with the College of Law, University of Arizona, Tucson, AZ 85721 and George A. Hughston, PhD, is affiliated with the Department of Family Resource and Human Development, Arizona State University, Tempe, AZ 85287.

163

arise in the functional abilities of any one part, the entire system will be affected to a greater or lesser extent. If the battery goes, a push-start may suffice, but if the starter motor is inoperable, the proposed trip will be canceled. The heart of family systems theory lies in its inclusion of all relationships as people interact with one another.

Family rules and guidelines assist with the description of each member's performance under proscribed conditions. The same principle of rules and guidelines may be applied to the psychotherapist in practice. The therapist temporarily becomes a part of the family system in order to assist in its movement toward more effective and satisfying activities. Greater awareness of intervening variables (parts influencing systemic operation) should provide the psychotherapist with increased alternatives for effective intervention.

Although specific information regarding the numbers of people cohabiting out-of-wedlock may be rather difficult to determine, few therapists would debate its increase among both the young and the old. In fact, benefits for the elderly may outweigh the benefits perceived by the young; especially if the cohabitation is not widely broadcast among extended family members. The range of elderly benefits from cohabitation may include greater retirement monies, lack of confrontation with children, fewer inheritance complications, simplified estate planning, etc. While family practitioners may be capable of presenting clients alternative assets and liabilities from a marriage and family perspective, few may be aware of the precise legal implications that could affect both cohabiting individuals and their families. Unfortunately, most of the more than 2.2 million cohabitors are unaware of the legal and financial consequences of their status. Serious problems frequently arise upon the death of one partner or when the couple decides to split up.

LEGAL IMPLICATIONS

This chapter outlines some very general legal realities of cohabitation for elderly people. The realities should be a part of systemic intervention with this clientele. *It cannot be overemphasized that legal counsel should be sought if the cohabitors have already acquired jointly owned property or commingled their money.* Psychotherapeutic obligations for effective client direction, however, are likewise unavoidable, as the law invades all areas of family life, and quite obviously affects the cohabiting older person. Although the elderly were socialized at a time when people were taught to be cautious in their business affairs, somehow that caution dissipates when they make a decision to cohabit. They have the mistaken belief that there will be no strings attached if they merely live together instead of marry.

The U.S. Supreme Court has recognized that people have the right of "intimate association" (Griswold vs. Connecticut, 1965). Laws affecting such association can nevertheless bring its citizens into line. It is economically beneficial to abide by the accepted social mores, traditions, etc., of our society. For instance, although the law does not in many places forbid cohabitation, nor does it actually enforce such laws where they do exist, certain legal ramifications can make such relationships undesirable due to the court's unwillingness to assist persons who are outside the law. These legal ramifications can take the form of a rule conditioning or eliminating some material benefit such as pension plans, inheritance, property ownership rights, welfare payments, or Social Security benefits.

Nevertheless, the law also protects our freedom to choose our intimates and to govern our day-to-day relations with them. This is more than an opportunity for the pleasures of self-expression, but is the foundation for the one responsibility among all others that most clearly defines our humanity (Karst, 1980).

When couples are married, the rights of the parties are governed by a formidable body of statutory or decisional law or by the increasingly common prenuptial agreement, so that the parties are easily aware of their rights or responsibilities (Gallen, 1981). Unlike marriage, which is favored in the eyes of the law, courts do not generally allow for the distribution of property jointly acquired during cohabitation. The law treats marriage as a partnership or joint venture between the parties, but does not accord such treatment to a nonmarried relationship, especially one that exists in the absence of a contract (Sack, 1987).

The intention of the parties is better decided at the beginning of a relationship rather than at its end. Once feelings and emotions have been injured and expectations of a wonderful union have dissipated, the original intentions of the parties, as to ownership of a substantial purchase or an alleged gift, may become the subject of a major lawsuit with all the accompanying legal fees.

Since unmarried cohabitation is legally a "form of association," giving rise to legal rights and potential obligations, it should also be entered into carefully. When there has been no written contract, a court will only look to the initial expectations of the parties in deciding the issues of the case; if one of the parties is deceased, the problems will be compounded. Entering such a relationship with some type of agreement may help, not only in the event of a dispute but also to prevent a dispute, by preserving the freedom of choice of the individuals involved.

AREAS OF CONCERN IN FAMILY PSYCHOTHERAPY

Although generalizations are risky in this area of law because individual state laws differ greatly, the following areas of concern can serve as foundational information for the therapist when discussing potential problems of cohabitation with his/her elderly clients:

First, it is better to enter an agreement in *advance* of actual cohabitation rather than to leave oneself open to the uncertainties of the law. Those who do not contract in advance may simply give the right to decide certain issues, such as property distribution, to an impartial court at a later time.

Second, state-by-state breakdowns are necessary so that the law of one jurisdiction can be separated from that of another, since even neighboring states have strikingly different rules of law as to property distribution within and without marriage (Gallen, 1981).

A typical question frequently asked is whether one cohabitor is liable for the debts incurred by his or her housemate. Generally, the answer would be "no," but a cohabitor can "assume" liability for certain of such debts by his or her actions; that is, if the persons have publicly held themselves as married or if the cohabitor had cosigned on charge card applications (Gallen, 1981).

Cohabitors live together at their own risk. An impartial judge or jury may be the final arbiters as to which person will be awarded control or ownership of a particular item of property. If there is no will specifically naming the cohabiting partner as a beneficiary, that person, under the law, may get nothing.

In his or her decision to allocate property, the judge will consider: (1) conduct of the parties; (2) subject matter of the purported agreement; and (3) the surrounding circumstances (to determine whether there was an agreement of partnership, joint venture, or some other tacit understanding between them or a written or oral trust).

When a written agreement is signed, the law presumes that the parties incorporated their true intentions into the contract. The instrument speaks for itself, and the courts will not hear testimony about understandings or discussions before the agreement was signed unless such information is necessary to interpret ambiguous terms.

As mentioned earlier, neither cohabitor is liable for the support of the other unless a contract or agreement was made between the parties. A court may imply the existence of an agreement of support, however, based upon the conduct and circumstances of their cohabitation. Generally speaking, liability for support of a cohabitor commences at zero and peaks to whatever the obligation would have been had the couple married. For those states still recognizing common law marriages, it is important that the couple try to avoid any public representations of marriage.

As in any contract, any and all agreements between the cohabitors should be in writing because those relying on oral contracts have a harder burden in proving their individual interpretation versus the other person's interpretation in the event of a conflict.

GUIDELINES FOR COHABITATION AGREEMENTS

Those wishing to draw up a cohabitation agreement should consult an attorney for final review. The couple would be well advised to draft a sample agreement prior to seeking legal counsel, thus reducing the amount of time the attorney will need to review their document. This can save the couple legal fees because they are not hassling over who should pay the vet bills or who will pay the dry cleaning expenses while the attorney's meter is ticking. Moreover, there may be problem areas the couple did not even know existed *until* wrestling with the details of an agreement.

The couple should consider the following in the draft agreement:

1. It should resemble a business partnership agreement; that is, the unmarried couple should state their intentions, and what it is that is being exchanged. (Sexual services cannot be exchanged or bargained for according to the infamous Lee Marvin "palimony" case) (Marvin vs. Marvin, 1981).
2. The agreement must be reasonable. One party cannot have the lion's share of benefits and the other get nothing in return. Similarly, what is being bargained for must be done without any duress, coercion, or undue influence.
3. The agreement must be comprehensive in that it covers every aspect of the relationship that could possibly be the subject of dispute in the event of a breakup. After the breakup is no time to try to make a reasonable assessment of what the parties intended at the onset of the relationship. At that point in time, it is unlikely that the two will agree on anything except, perhaps, the belief that each had been "taken" by the other.

In the early glow of an intimate relationship, there may be considerable resistance to completing a detailed cohabitation agreement. Some couples object to the contract approach because they feel it is unromantic, and that their newly formed relationship should not be hampered at its inception with mutual suspicion. Those romantically involved may not want to think that there will ever by any problems or that they may be taken advantage of in the future. However, without an advance agreement, these fears of future heartache might well become a self-fulfilling prophecy. Or defining the scope of the relationship in business form (written agreement) could appear as a legal obligation and indirectly seem to imply that the responsibility for one another's welfare is produced by duty and not love. Further, if circumstances change, it may be feared that the contract could restrict the ability to allow for the change, removing the element of desired flexibility every relationship needs and wants to have.

While these objections may have some validity, the likelihood of the agreement making their future more pleasant by affirming responsible self-care and thus moderating the fear of the unknown may outweigh such concerns.

There are five key areas that the therapist and his or her clients should be aware of when considering the overall relationship system: (1) whether cohabitation is legal in their state; (2) whether there is an agreement, expressed or implied, that indicates a support obligation of one of the cohabitors to the other; (3) the status of property that had been acquired by one of the parties prior to the cohabitation or during its inception, as most states hold that property acquired before the unmarried relationship began remains with the true (original) owner; (4) the "ownership of property acquired during the relationship" (most states will look to see in whose name ownership has been recorded or titled and how the cohabitors wanted to allocate their jointly-appropriated property); and (5) the presence of a will. (Every state allows a person at his or her death to distribute real and personal property as he or she chooses. Here there is no difference between married and unmarried couples. Sometimes, however, a cohabitor's legacy must fail, in whole or in part, due to the legally superior claims of a surviving spouse or children of the former/current marriage.)

If a person dies without a will, each state provides a particular disposition of the estate depending on who the survivors are and how they are related to the decedent. Cohabitors are not part of that distribution.

A word of caution: The claims of an unmarried cohabitor, even if substantiated by written agreement, can be subordinated to claims of the decedent's surviving parent(s) and sibling(s). Unless there is a valid will, children may sometimes get the entire proceeds of an estate, or, if a spouse survives, the estate will be divided among the previous (legal) family alone and *not* the surviving cohabitor.

Unmarried cohabitors should draft a will because if they do not, state law will determine who receives the decedent's property and in what proportion. This would usually mean that a relative of the decedent, rather than the cohabitor, would receive the decedent's assets. It could also mean that, if no blood relatives could be located, the assets would be escheated to the state. The will is independent of any written agreement the cohabitors may have drafted.

In other words, if one cohabitor dies without a will, the other cohabitor has no "automatic" inheritance rights absent a written agreement. If there is a written agreement providing for support, the survivor could claim, as a creditor, against the estate of the deceased. But such a written agreement transferring property to, or the continuing support of the unmarried survivor is extremely difficult to enforce as a matter of law, and administrators of the estate are very likely to be uncooperative.

Along with a will, cohabitors should consider purchasing insurance for one another. Individual states have different criteria for cohabitors so the couple must be candid and explain their situation to their insurance agent when purchasing insurance protection.

A cohabitor cannot assign his or her rights to receive Social Security benefits to the other since federal law allows only "spouses" the right to receive such benefits. However, a cohabitor can assign his or her right to receive pension benefits *if* the express language of the pension contract allows it.

Similarly, a cohabitor may be able to receive Workmen's Compensation benefits under the account of his or her deceased partner if the particular jurisdiction allows it. Some states permit the awarding of death benefits to a surviving unmarried cohabitor if the cohabitor can prove his or her dependency on the deceased for the "necessaries of life," and prove he or she was living with the decedent at the time of death. Receipt of this particular benefit is a prime example of why an attorney should be consulted. An attorney will know the particular law of the state where the agreement is being drafted and could make a provision for such a death benefit allowance if the matter is brought to his or her attention at its inception.

A lawsuit is a costly last resort; it exposes the personal life of the couple to public scrutiny as well as the scrutiny of a judge and a jury. It also requires a court to decide a matter that could and should have been settled by an agreement between the cohabiting couples during the life of their relationship.

REFERENCES

Barton, C. (1986). Cohabitation contracts: Extramarital partnerships and law reform. London: Gower Publishing Co. Ltd.

Gallen, R., Kaplan, J., & Bianco, J. (1981). *The unmarried couple's legal handbook*. New York: Dell.

Griswold v. Connecticut, 381 U.S. 479 (1965).

Karst, K. L. (1980). The freedom of intimate association. *89 Yale Law Jour*, 624-92.

Marvin v. Marvin, 122 Cal. App. 3rd 871, 176 Cal. Rptr. 555 (1981).

Sack, S. M. (1987). *The complete legal guide to marriage, divorce, custody, and living together*. New York: McGraw-Hill.

APPENDIX

Items to consider at the onset of the relationship;
1. Legal status. Learn how the law in your state treats common law marriage and cohabitation.
2. Statement of the purpose of the contract. Will it create an equal relationship between the parties or will one party be dominant while the other passive?
3. Legality of the agreement. Is it intended to be legally binding or merely a statement of expectations?
4. Names of the parties and their ages, financial conditions, states of health, etc.
5. Aims of the parties (collective and individual goals). Companionship, financial support, etc.?
6. Duration of agreement. Expectation to last a lifetime, a specific period, or until a specified event occurs?
7. Employment/retirement decisions. Who wants or can work, and what priorities or sacrifices will be made toward that goal?
8. Income and expense issues. How much income is available? How is it to be treated? Pooled? What about savings?
9. Prior property issues (that held by each at the inception of the relationship). Name what property each owns and what it consists of (real and/or personal). How is that property to be treated — shared? separate?
10. Property acquired during cohabitation. Will it be shared? treated like community property? Who is to manage or have control over the property? How will joint gifts be treated in case of a split up? Get a receipt when you contribute money toward the purchase of property or assets that will be used by both cohabitants.
11. Life insurance policies. Who are the named beneficiaries?
12. Pension funds. Who are beneficiaries? What does their state allow for unmarried couples?
13. Debts. List what each one currently owes for both joint and separate purchases. Also consider individual attitudes toward credit; does one abhor credit while the other thrives on it?
14. Living arrangements. Where to live? Location? Type of dwelling?

15. Treatment of family and or guests in their mutual home.
16. Household tasks, how will they be divided up?
17. Change of surname of the female cohabitor?
18. Sexual behavior. Monogamous? Rules for disclosure if open to other relationships?
19. Personal habits. Smoking, hobbies, need for privacy?
20. Monetary relationships with other family members, financial obligations?
21. Wills. Upon death, how will property be distributed? Will each draft a will leaving each other property? Prepare a will to accurately reflect your desires, not only as to the cohabitation but all other devisees.
22. Rental contract issues. Protect yourself whenever you move into an apartment or cooperative by:
    A. getting both names on the lease (person who signs lease is the lawful tenant),
    B. signing a residence agreement with your cohabitant,
    C. documenting your intentions with other evidence (let each person pay the rent at different times to show both are responsible for the lease of the apartment and for the utility bills. This demonstrates that the partners had an implied contract to share in the proceeds if the apartment should be converted into a cooperative. Save all receipts.
23. Avoid making promises you do not intend to keep or may not be able to keep.
24. Speak to an experienced lawyer if you believe you have been victimized.
25. Be aware that concurrent marital status will create more difficulty in being recognized in court, especially if one or both of the cohabitants are still legally married to someone else. Adultery does not get a "seal of approval" as a result of cohabitant status (Barton, 1986).

Older Families and Issues of Alcohol Misuse: A Neglected Problem in Psychotherapy

Eloise Rathbone-McCuan
Jacquelyn Hedlund

SUMMARY. This article addresses some of the recent information that has been collected on the issues of alcohol misuse in later stages of the life span. It discusses the risks to both long-term alcoholics who have grown old with their drinking problem and the issues facing those persons for whom the risks of alcohol become apparent in later life. Three cases are included to illustrate the different consequences of alcoholism in the family as it impacts on separate members and generations within the family system. Authors discuss some principles of intervention and prevention that can and should be applied by different mental health and health practitioners that work with older persons and their family groups.

INTRODUCTION

This article presents an overview of alcohol abuse among the elderly and discusses what is known about the psycho-social-physical factors associated with late-life abuse. Three cases illustrate how the problems of alcohol may impact on the multi-generational family. Authors review use of various clinical interventions to assist

Eloise Rathbone-McCuan, PhD, MSW, is affiliated with the College of Education and Social Services, University of Vermont, Burlington, VT 05405. Jacquelyn Hedlund, MPH, is affiliated with the College of Medicine, University of Vermont, Burlington, VT 05405. Her participation in this project was completed in conjunction with a Medical Student Geriatric Fellowship from the National Council on Aging and Travelers Insurance Company.

173

the older alcoholic and other family members applying a general social systems perspective of psychotherapy and counseling.

OVERVIEW OF ALCOHOL PROBLEMS AMONG THE AGED

The epidemiological research on alcohol use and misuse among the elderly is problematic. National surveys of drinking in the general adult population have *not* produced accurate rates of heavy drinking or problematic consumption patterns generalizable to the elderly. Surveys of drinking practices among the elderly tend to produce more reliable rates for older men than older women because alcoholism among women, irrespective of their age, is a more hidden problem.

Williams (1984) summarized the problems of survey methods as a means of detecting alcoholism among the aged. Estimates indicate that 12 to 15 million Americans are alcohol dependent or in some stage of alcoholism. Up to 35 million more people are estimated to be affected indirectly. The elderly are projected to have alcohol abuse rates of between two and ten percent. Meyers et al. (1985) commented on the growing concern about the potential to distort the estimates through assumptions of too much or too little problem drinking. Estimate variance speaks to the need for better research tools, more clinical case studies, detailed assessments of the co-existence of health, social, and psychological problems, and exploration of treatment. Incorrect assumptions about alcohol abuse patterns contribute to stereotypes of the skid row and homeless older person as alcoholic.

The problems of the alcoholic grown are recognized more frequently than those of the "late-on-set" problem drinker who develops drinking risks in later life. These two patterns of abuse may create different problems requiring different interventions. Some older alcoholics have a history of unsuccessful treatment encounters with periods of sobriety that cannot be sustained. Others have never been involved in any formal or informal treatment because of personal denial. Denial, operating as a key factor in the dependency process, is a major barrier to help-seeking. For the elderly it is a problem reinforced by the stigma of alcohol that is especially great among older women. Also, it is a problem that is reinforced by others who fail to recognize the alcohol related issues or who remain silent and try to protect the older alcoholic.

Professionals often misdiagnosis the problems of alcoholism considering it to be a symptom of cognitive deterioration or depression, however, these can be associated with alcohol intoxication, other forms of drug dependency, depression, or a combination. Family members may associate some of the emotional and behavioral dynamics of alcoholism with other conditions and may dismiss them as "just part of the process of growing old and getting senile." To engage the older person in help-seeking there must be a bridge between the individual and the sources of recovery assistance, but in too many cases that bridge is not readily available from social peers, family members or professionals. This leaves the older alcoholic with the potential of being very isolated and vulnerable.

The disruptive impact of alcoholism is felt no matter what generation of family member is alcohol dependent. To understand the various problem patterns as they impact differently on each generation, several case illustrations are included as a framework.

The Marshall Family

The Marshall household was a three generational family unit. An aged father, George, lived with his middle-aged daughter Patty, her husband, and three teenage grandchildren. His difficulty adjusting to the death of his wife and living alone lead to the invitation for him to live with Patty's family. George became very involved with his grandchildren to supplement the limited time of working parents and initially it was a benefit to the family so George felt of value to those he loved. This family encountered what Pittman (1987) describes as a crisis "out-of-the-blue" when Scott, the oldest grandchild, entered what the family first called a "teenage personality change." He was involved in heavy peer drinking and became very aggressive and hostile to his family. The hostile behavior caused intense conflict that was most visible between George and Scott. Before alcohol abuse was recognized, his grandfather attempted to reprimand Scott each time his behavior became too aggressive. When George learned from his daughter that she was sure that Scott had an alcohol problem, George felt that harsh measures must be taken and he prescribed "throwing him out of the house until he learned to behave himself."

George did not know about adolescent alcoholism or how to express his concern about Scott and the conflicts between husband and wife. Even after Scott entered a program for teenage chemical dependents, George felt isolated from his family and blamed himself for not preventing Scott's problem. At the point George was deciding to leave the family without an idea of where to go, Scott's primary alcoholism counselor convinced all the family to enter therapy. The counseling helped George reestablish his relationship with Scott and improved the communication throughout the family.

The Patterson Family

Elizabeth, a healthy, active 82-year-old widow, was closely connected to her three children and their families. Her busy life was filled with travel and visitations with each family, but this was interrupted by a heart attack. During her year of "slowing down and taking care of herself" she had very limited contact with Daniel, her youngest son, and his family who were becoming embroiled in the pathology of alcoholism. She knew of the serious conflict, but lacked any knowledge of Dan's extensive drinking problem. When Dan called to ask if he could move in with her, she was more than willing if this would help his marriage get back on track. Dan had gone to Alcoholics Anonymous and had been sober for a short period, but then he began an affair with an alcoholic woman that produced a demand from his wife to leave their home. At the point Dan moved, his children were devastated and afraid and his wife was angry that Elizabeth was siding against her by letting Dan into her home. As Dan plunged into alcoholic interactions with his mistress, conflict increased between Elizabeth and Dan's wife. Because Dan lived with her, she had opportunities to observe his alcoholic binges and hurtful behaviors to the family. As the situation worsened, she decided that she must seek the advice of her other two children. Both children were very direct about the importance of Elizabeth starting to attend Al-Non. She and her closest friend went to Al-Non and received support and guidance about how to relate to Dan and to understand the family crises. Several months later Dan's wife and children entered family counseling and through Elizabeth's continued participation in Al-Non she was able to receive much needed support and to give support to Dan's family as they confronted the alcoholism.

The Printer Family

Margaret Printer was a 68-year-old retired widow living in senior housing because her husband's death made it impossible to afford their small home. Her two married sons lived on opposite coasts and were in regular, however limited, contact with Margaret except when they made an annual visit. Her adjustment to being alone was difficult because of limited transportation and losing daily access to her close neighbors and friends. While these friendships were maintained with phone calls, she missed the face-to-face interaction. Because she was one of the youngest residents in the complex, she did not make friends with the elderly tenants. Lack of social contact changed when she was invited to be a member of a daily card game with some of the younger women in her building. Each day the game would be conducted over cocktails and over several months of regular games, Margaret began to drink three or four drinks at each game — her "social drinking" was becoming a dependency.

The increased drinking began to interrupt her daily eating and exercise, but Margaret was involved in active denial of alcohol dependency. Because of the infrequent contact with her sons, they were unaware of alcohol abuse and thought their mother sounded depressed during phone conversations. Because of their "nagging," she saw her family doctor, however, she did not discuss her increased alcohol consumption before starting to use a prescribed anti-depressant. The combined use of alcohol and the anti-depressant produced an unintentional overdose requiring her emergency hospitalization. When one of the sons arrived at the hospital he met with the medical social worker who explained that Margaret had required detoxification and then transfer to the substance abuse treatment unit. He was hostile at an implication of his mother's alcohol dependency and he facilitated her decision to leave the treatment program. When Margaret got back to the housing complex and the son returned home, she became afraid for her own safety and sought help from the residential social worker. The social worker suggested that she begin to attend a counseling group for older people sponsored by the mental health center. Through the therapeutic processes available in the group, Margaret was quickly connected into a senior peer alcoholism program.

INDIVIDUAL AND GROUP
THERAPEUTIC INTERVENTIONS

There is little information about the use of family-centered therapy for the treatment of alcoholism among the elderly and how the older nonalcoholic person can become involved in therapeutic processes. These cases provide information about common dynamics drawing the family into the elder's alcohol problems and illustrate the impact on the quality of family relationships because of some other member's alcoholism.

More communities are developing services for older people with drug dependencies and within these programs intervention can be either age-specific, that is, programs are designed to provide outreach and treatment to only older people or they are adult-general. In the latter type of programs, there are special services introduced for the different needs of older people. Some of the life-stage modifications and adaptations include (1) special outreach programs concentrating on settings where groups of older people live such as senior citizen housing or retirement communities, (2) involvement of older recovered alcoholics used for peer counseling with special sensitivities to social, emotional, and health needs of older people with alcohol problems, (3) extended programs for inpatient detoxification providing medical monitoring and treatment for other related physical problems, (4) transportation supports to enable seniors to get to group therapy and counseling sessions, and (5) service referral networks coordinating health, substance abuse, and senior citizen service networks.

It is the consensus among experienced practitioners that insight-oriented individual counseling may be less effective, overall, than group treatment. When individual counseling is utilized it takes on a more active orientation to environmental factors as compared to traditional psychotherapy with younger or middle-aged adults. For example, Margaret Printer was endangered by alcohol abuse as the result of a complex cluster of grief and social isolation factors. If a counselor were to utilize an insight approach, recommended after the individual has stopped drinking, the focus of therapy would include exploring the unresolved emotional and social issues of widowhood. The practitioner would also engage in identifying community resources and encourage the older client to participate in those services as needed.

Mrs. Printer was forced to give up her home, and move to a strange residential environment resulting in a loss of contact with important friends not easily replaced with an intimate support system. With eagerness, she became part of a clique of women interacting around alcohol consumption. As is true of many late-onset problem drinkers, there was no advanced knowledge of the risks of alcohol dependency. For some older people with histories of social drinking, companionship that involves the use of alcohol may start out as an acceptable alternative to being alone. They do not question the norms of drinking behavior and proceed to increase their own consumption.

In situations such as this not all older people will become alcohol dependent. Some may evaluate the social dynamics in the relationships and decide *not* to continue interactions with the network of heavy drinkers and they proceed to find alternative social relationships. For others, the drive to experience regular and predictable social contact dominates over caution about the behavior patterns. Isolated older people will participate in a social milieu of heavy drinking with or without knowledge that their own alcohol dependency may be increasing. When dealing with the factors of social isolation and alcohol abuse, the counselor needs to assess these relationships and support the individual to develop alternatives networks that reduce risks of alcohol dependency (Rathbone-McCuan and Hashimi, 1982).

Some of the principles applied in adult group alcoholism therapy are applicable to the older population, for example, homogeneity of group members. Older people in recovery may feel that being in a group with younger people is very difficult because life events, circumstances, and personal priorities vary with life stage. Job-related risks encountered by younger people have little application to their lives as retired individuals. The concerns that older people have about health and safety associated with alcohol abuse are not necessarily as important to younger people who do not perceive physical risks as relevant as economic or career threats.

Sometimes the informal structure of a group, even less structured than an AA group, can be useful for outreach when an individual is exploring personal issues of drug dependency. Group leaders do not necessarily have to be trained alcoholism counselors to offer a social contact that helps the older person take steps to address alcohol issues. Some group socialization programs for aged, such as those available in senior citizen centers, have referral linkages to formal and informal sources of alcohol treatment. Also, many older problem drinkers benefit from participating in multiple groups, each offering another source of socialization not dependent on alcohol consumption. Unfilled and unrewarding social time is dangerous for older problem drinkers because it perpetuates the conditions in which they are most likely to abuse alcohol.

TREATMENT IN THE FAMILY CONTEXT

The Marshall and Patterson cases illustrate how alcohol abuse touches the lives of older people who are not abusers. Families go through many traumatic experiences prior to realizing alcohol-related problems. One member may challenge other members who deny the problem and this leads to further denial and anger within the family system. There is, however, a difference between denial behavior and a lack of knowledge about the stages and dynamics of alcohol dependency. While information is not always enough to prevent denial, without information many family members are handicapped in facing the issue.

When assessing values and norms of the nuclear family, there are fewer people whose values must be understood as the group is conceptualized as a smaller unit. If the practitioner expands the family system to an extended multigenerational group, she should be prepared for the possibility of greater value diversity and conflict. Since all value differences cannot be addressed in the course of short-term intervention, it is important to identify the most important sources of conflict surrounding the alcoholism. The therapist must know which family members assume the most important roles in the transference and countertransference with the alcoholic member(s).

The intervention received by the Patterson family was through a combination of formal therapy and informal self-help. The decision to not involve Elizabeth in the counseling with the nuclear family was justified because she had found her own source of support through Al-Non, but if she had not made this connection she would have been assisted greatly by participation in the family therapy process. When to draw an older family member such as Elizabeth into the counseling process must be judged according to their position and interactional processes with the alcoholic member. The addition of individual counseling and supplemental group therapy for specific family members can also be helpful. The practitioner must not overload the family with too much therapy from too many sources unless the family has the energy to cope with different therapeutic relationships, the economic means to cover therapy costs, and receives professional assistance to coordinate services needed by the different generations.

The vulnerability of elderly people to the consequences of alcoholic family members can be great, for instance, where the elderly person is dependent upon care and assistance from a family member who is alcoholic. The caregiver's physical, social, economic, and psychological capacity to perform caregiving functions may be greatly reduced by drinking, thus, leaving the elder neglected, abused, or exploited. In cases where there is physical risk to the elder because of the caregiver's substance abuse, it may be necessary for the elderly person to have a protective advocate who offers interventions to protect the elder from the alcoholic caregiver.

If the dependent elder is the alcoholic receiving care from nonalcoholic family members, a different set of dynamics arises. As more caregivers are joining self-help support groups to enable them to cope with the stress of long-term home care, there is awareness of how alcoholism complicates the caregiving. Many caregivers have chronic alcoholic parents from whom they once separated and if called upon to re-enter that parent's life will experience re-engagement with the pain and fear of the alcoholism. Children of aged alcoholics are especially vulnerable to these dynamics in heavy caregiving situations because it brings into play earlier patterns of control and manipulation. Adult children of aged alcoholics may need to separate, again, from the destructiveness of the parent's alcoholism in the face of conflicting guilt about the parent's condition. In these situations, a decision not to assume the caregiver role because of personal costs should be supported in therapy. Supportive counseling can help to reach that decision and to act upon it without placing the dependent elder at-risk because their care is neglected.

Community professionals can serve a gatekeeper function to assist the older person into treatment. In those situations where it is the older person who has the abuse problem, health and social service professionals may be in an excellent position to identify the abuse and act to promote help-seeking. For older people, physicians are the most typical source of regular professional contact and may be the only person with sufficient contact to prompt help-seeking. Unfortunately, too many physicians and social workers miss or avoid opportunities to engage their older patients around substance dependency. Most clinicians have completed their education without learning about alcoholism and its prevention. With training, physicians and social workers can educate older persons about the negative effects of alcohol on existing health problems, its contributory role in other diseases, and inform them about the potential misuse of alcohol with prescribed drugs. Dual dependency is a common problem confronting the late-life problem drinker because of the multiple medications taken for medical problems without knowledge of risks.

Professionals need to know how to confront the issue of alcohol misuse in ways that increase problem recognition. Effective confrontation involves a combination of reality about behaviors and risks as well as support of the individual's ability to act in their self-interest for sobriety. One of the best opportunities to introduce confrontation is immediately after a medical or interpersonal crisis that has involved drinking. This may be a time when the individual is more receptive to a referral. When a professional makes a referral she must be willing to take the time required for making an appropriate and complete contact based on knowledge of community resources. The most readily available source of assistance is Alcoholics Anonymous (AA), but this may not be the appropriate source if very serous physical and psychological problems are also present. Inpatient programs, even if they are not specialized for a geriatric population, may be the best source with sufficient health care and medical supports. In the referral process, the practitioner must know how to engage the family to encourage their cooperation and coordination in rehabilitation.

CONCLUSION

As issues of family life and the aging process become more prevalent in this society, it is essential to recognize the range of stresses that may confront families. It is a misconception to view most family crises as having no impact on the eldest members. Conversely, many of the predictable events and circumstances of aging, especially those associated with losses of resources and independence, can provoke family crises. Alcohol related abuse has the power to create much hurt within and across generations as it is difficult if not impossible to put protective boundaries around the fear, anger, and loss of people's trust and faith in each other generated by alcohol abuse. Older people may drag their alcoholism along with each passing year until they reach old age or they may encounter its power only after they have journeyed throughout their adult life without experiencing its full risk. Their family, whether it be spouses, siblings, children or grandchildren, will find themselves caught in the rhythms of the "drunken dance." As the field of family psychotherapy forms new approaches to treat the psychosocial needs of older and multigenerational families, the problems of alcoholism will surface in the dynamics of those family systems.

When the alcohol abuser is the eldest family member, that individual should enjoy the same access to potential recovery available to a younger family member. If the older person is one of the family members suffering from the consequences of some other member's dependency, then they should be a focus of as much concern as other younger members. It is essential that family therapists and alcoholism counselors develop the competencies needed to help families and older individuals when they are ready to take steps to pursue greater levels of individual and collective well-being through the management of alcohol abuse in their lives.

REFERENCES

Meyers, A.R., Hingson, R., Mucatel, M., Heerin, T., and Goldman, E. (1985). The social epidemiology of alcohol use by urban older adults. *International Journal of Aging and Human Development*, 21, 49-59.

Pittman, F.S. (1987). *Turning Points: Treating Families in Transition and Crisis*. New York: W.W. Norton.

Rathbone-McCuan, E. and Hashimi, J. (1982). *Isolated Elders*. Rockville: Aspen Systems.

Williams, M. (1984). Alcohol and the elderly: An overview. *Alcohol, Health and Research World*, 8, 3-9.

The Burden of Insight:
A Basis for Constructive Response

Victor A. Christopherson

SUMMARY. The nature of insight is explored with regard to its significance in interpersonal relationships within the family context containing an adult caregiver child and one or more elderly parents. The burden of insight derives from the assumption of the responsibilities congruent with insight. While the burden is most often assumed by the adult child, the principal caregiver, it is relevant, also, for the therapist as well as the recipient of the care. The article discusses the significance of the burden of insight with regard to two major causes of family disequilibration, generational differences and the decrements of senescence.

> Can a blind man lead a blind man?
> Will they not both fall into a pit?
>
> (Luke 6:39)

Insight yields perspective, and perspective may well be a mixed blessing. On the one hand, perspective facilitates the resolution of interpersonal problems, but on the other, it dissolves the comforting shroud of innocence. Once innocence is gone, the individual must assume full responsibility for his or her behavior. Mistakes may still be made, but they are now made in the interest of or efforts toward positive goal-directed behavior. Such mistakes can be corrected as experience and evaluation accrue.

In families, the parents are assumed and expected to understand the nature and behavior of the child, and they have been given the charge of responsibility for the welfare and care of all offspring. We

---

Victor A. Christopherson, EdD, is Professor, Family Studies, The University of Arizona, Tucson, AZ 85721.

185

know that this is an imperfect assumption, and, unfortunately, the instances of parental ineptitude and mistreatment of children are legion. In general, however, no better alternative to parental care has been found.

Parental responsibility for the care, welfare, and socialization of children has generations, even centuries, of more-or-less successful tradition behind it. Now what happens when the situation is reversed? Children assume the caregiving responsibilities for their elderly parents. There is little successful tradition in the United States to serve as a reliable guideline for either parent or child in this turn of events. In the case of grown children assuming the role of parent to their own elderly parents, the path is often uncharted and murky. When insight is absent in such a situation, perspective falters, problems begin to cluster, and various degrees of despair result.

Insight, like love, is something everyone knows something about. Also, like love, it is somewhat difficult to define. Its meaning tends to change as situations change. Davidson and Sternberg (1986) define insight as the sifting out of relevant from irrelevant information, the process of assembling apparently unrelated facts in a coherent way, and charting a course of action taking the facts or pattern of facts into account. Bohm (1981) states that insight is primarily an inward perception, one seen through the mind rather than the eyes. Anna Freud's statement concerning insight, however, may well be the most fruitful for our purpose. She writes, "Insight takes a person further in his/her capacity for understanding than is otherwise the case" (1981).

Some years ago, Willard Waller (1951) revealed a certain insight of his own when he described what he called "the principle of least interest." The upshot of the concept was that the individual in a relationship who was the least emotionally involved, or had the least interest in maintaining the relationship, controlled it. The one who was most committed, or had the greatest emotional investment, would make the greatest compromises or concessions in order to maintain the relationship. The "burden of insight," in a sense, works just the other way around. The individual with the most insight into the dynamics of a relationship, has the burden or responsibility to do what is necessary to maintain and facilitate it. In addition, insight, unlike emotional involvement, is based on knowledge. Knowledge and insight, however, are not synonymous nor are they equivalent. As Bohm (1981) writes, "The intense energy of insight is what can dissolve all kinds of blocks and barriers, including those responsible for self-centeredness." Knowledge, per se, seldom accomplishes this.

INSIGHT AND ADJUSTMENT

The contexts in which adjustment takes place are of vital importance. One might well have a good deal of insight in one context but very little in another. One such context is the family, the most basic primary group. Primary group relationships, like larger patterns of cultural behavior, appear to evolve without conscious intent. The productive patterns tend to survive, while the nonproductive ones largely fall by the wayside. In short, they do not always depend upon the participating individuals' awareness and conscious intent. Their success is largely because of their adaptive significance. Insight, however, is a conscious attribute, and depends on an awareness of the behavioral dynamics involved in a relationship. When the time-tested relationships sustain new elements that cast former patterns of reciprocal behavior into untested or new ground, it is essential not only that at least one party to the relationship understand the nature and probable cause of the change, but that he or she assume the responsibility for guiding the relationship in positive directions. This responsibility is the basis of the burden of insight.

When the situation involves adult children acting as caregivers for their elderly parents, insight can be a double-edged sword. While there is no doubt that it is helpful for the adult child to understand the nature and implications of the changes that accompany senescence, realistically, assuming the consequent burdens for maintaining optimal conditions within the limits of available resources can be an awesome task.

That such an application of insight does not always occur is very evident. The very nature of the concept of "burden" is one that suggests people often try to avoid burdens rather than assume them if choice is possible. Unless, however, the burden is assumed by the individual with insight, the basis of disturbed or disequilibrated interpersonal relationships within the family can increase and intensify to the point where there seems little hope of positive resolution. The parties to the relationship are caught up in a pattern of reaction instead of positive action. At this point, where neither insight nor the assumption of responsibility for positive steps toward bettering the situation is in evidence, it might well be necessary for therapeutic intervention by a professional to be brought into play.

Fortunately, insight is not a basic "given" that one either has or does not have. It is a quality that can be developed and subsequently utilized. The most productive role of the therapist in a multigenerational family situation that has become reactive and hostile, might well be the generation of insight, particularly on the part of the adult child, and in the elderly parent if possible. If the therapist can help the adult child attain insight and perspective, much will have been accomplished.

Sometimes information and knowledge alone will bring about insight. Other times, overcoming barriers and resistance will be a part of the problem. The willingness to assume the burden for bettering things is not always easily achieved. The burden of insight must be shouldered with a measure of perspective in order to maintain a healthy balance. Complete selflessness can lead to such sacrificial behavior that everyone suffers, including self, other family members, and the elderly parents as well. When adult children do too much, too soon, and too often for their parents, it becomes reminiscent of Freud's "reaction formation" mechanism. In this case, the destruction of the parents is accomplished unwittingly by rendering them helpless and dependent through the provision of too much assistance. Most often, however, the problems lie in the other direction. Needed, in order to restore equilibrium to disturbed relationships, is often little more than an extra measure of patience and tolerance. The decrements of senescence can be irritating to adult caregivers if they are not familiar with the patterns and processes. Occasionally, however, when the changes transcend the bounds of the normal, such as in the organic brain syndromes, Alzheimer's or Pick's diseases, the burdens can become immense. Insight is needed in such circumstances to objectify available courses of action in order to preserve self, family and resources. Sacrificial altruism in such cases is of little value to anyone and can be the antithesis of insightful behavior.

PROBLEM SOURCES

While problems that afflict multigenerational families are abundant, two principal sources which, when understood, yield insight, stem from the sequelae of senescence per se, and from the differential perspectives of generations; i.e., cohort differences. There are many other sources to be sure, but these two general and broad categories account for much of the grief experienced by families with adult children and elderly parents.

GENERATIONAL PERSPECTIVES

No attempt is made here to characterize cohort perspectives as such. Rather, the point to be made is that unless the key individual, or the one upon whom the burden of insight principally falls, is aware of the general nature of differential cohort perspective, misunderstandings and faulty motive attributions can easily occur.

Ruth Benedict (1938) a number of years ago wrote about cultural discontinuities. She called attention to the discontinuous nature of a child, socialized as a child, suddenly becoming a parent and having to switch perspectives. The adult child appears to be in a doubly discontinuous situation having had to make the adjustment from child to parent, still being a child to one's elderly parent, and then having to assume parent-like roles in relation to the elderly parent. If this sounds complicated, it is.

The elderly parent, meanwhile, assuming reasonably good health, is striving to maintain independence and also to enjoy the situation of being cared "about." At the same time, the parent may well need to be "cared for." Perspectives can become confused and motive attribution distorted. It is difficult for both generations to sort things out. Insight is needed, and it can often be brought to bear best by someone who has the larger view and has "been there" before; i.e., the practitioner or therapist. Insight, by way of emphasis, is only part of the scenario. It is important for the practitioner to keep in mind that understanding the dynamics in which the family is caught up is only the beginning. It is also necessary to bring about the assumption of the burden that accompanies the insight if the situation is to improve measurably. If this can be managed, the result should be much like the outcome suggested by Erikson (1964)

> . . . the parent dealing with a child will be strengthened in "his" vitality, in "his" sense of identity, and in "his" readiness for ethical action by the very ministrations by means of which "he" secures to the child vitality, future identity, and eventual readiness for ethical action. (p. 232)

In short, the person who may be seemingly inconvenienced by having to act in such a way as to keep the aged parent's welfare in mind, nevertheless has his or her own self-economy strengthened in the process because the act is one of choice and understanding. Lewis and Lewis (1986) suggest several areas of intergenerational conflict in which such insight is extremely beneficial. They are: independence versus dependence, morality versus mortality, integration versus isolation, optimism versus pessimism, and resolution versus dissolution.

The issue in independence versus dependence is the acceptance by the adult child of the perspective that the parent is trying to maintain independence but, in fact, is becoming increasingly more dependent. Also, the adult child must accept the fact of the parent's diminishing capacities, and that the aged parent can no longer fulfill the child's own need to be parented in some sense. Once such a perspective is internalized and accepted, the adult child can make the necessary allowances and can do what is necessary to facilitate harmony in the relationship.

The morality versus mortality issue is an acceptance of the fact that the parent is eventually going to die in spite of any or all of the ministrations dictated by society and conscience to keep the aged member alive and well. This recognition brings with it a sense of one's own mortality. The conflict between society's expectations and one's own honest inclinations can result in guilt or expressed anger. Insight into the dynamics of the relationship can attenuate the discomfort and prevent the anger from being displaced onto other innocent members in the family context. The source of the negative feelings, once recognized and properly dealt with, clears the way for planned and constructive action as indicated.

The issue in the integration versus isolation problem is the feeling on the part of the adult child that his or her own adjustment to the demands of life is being threatened by the additional demands of the aged parent. Lewis and Lewis (1986) suggest that the adult child fears the demands of the parent will force abandonment or isolation from the social, economic and religious patterns, and relationships that the child deems important and necessary in his/her own life space. Not infrequently, care of elderly parents within the home calls for decisions that might, to the outsider, seem a bit harsh or unfeeling. For example, should an aged parent become increasingly demanding of the time and attention of the adult child, to the extent, in fact, that the demands become unreasonable, the child must have the insight to understand the cause, achieve the perspective, and make some decisions that preserve the family tranquility. The decisions might be to place the parent in a long-term care facility or to leave the parent, as frequently as necessary, in order to pursue interests and relationships with others, or in some other fashion to be firm and reasonable in the relationship with the parent. Insight of this nature helps prevent guilt and self-pity that otherwise could easily result.

The adult child must be able to maintain an essential optimism about the future in the face of the parent's sometimes pessimistic view that life is about over, and there is little to look forward to. The burden of insight in this context is to take the life cycle into account both for the parent and for self. Acceptance of one's place in the life cycle in a firm and realistic manner helps prevent confusion between the implications for the two generations. Even though aged parents may be starkly realistic concerning "tomorrow," the adult child should be able to distinguish his/her own future in clear enough fashion that grace and forbearance can be brought to bear.

A final note concerning generational differences is that it is of utmost importance to realize that different points of view concerning many of the values and events of life derive from the normal cultural changes that accrue with the passage of time. It is even more crucial, however, to express such insight in a willingness to make allowances for these differences in the form of tolerance and understanding. Christ called it "going the second mile." When such allowances can be expressed with perspective and without guilt or remorse, the burden has been shouldered.

Another context in which the burden of insight must be levied, is that of dealing with the process of senescence or the normal changes that occur as a concomitant of aging.

SENESCENCE

The three principal levels at which the process of aging affects the adult caregiver child are the physical or biological, the mental or cognitive, and the emotional.

At the physical or biological level, the diminishing strength and constitutional capacities of the aged parent will likely place additional demands on the time, energy and patience of the adult child. Perhaps as often as not, the aged parent will insist on performing the activities or chores in question beyond the point where his/her waning capacities will permit goal attainment without generating frustration or alarm on the part of observers. Care has to be taken not to jump in and prematurely deprive the parent of important prerogatives that, in fact, the elderly parent can assume given a little extra time or task redefinition. On the other hand, when the parent cannot adequately perform the task, or when a genuine parental reluctance becomes apparent, a new solution must be found. In either case, insight into the senescence process usually places the burden of the major adjustment on the shoulders of the adult child. The adult child must expand the base of his or her own roles, others must be brought into the process, or the task must be modified or eliminated in some fashion. The important thing is that whatever action is taken, it be done free of guilt, blame, or undue remorse. In short, it becomes simply a practical solution to the changing situation. When the insight is shared or reciprocal, of course, the entire process is facilitated.

Various types of sensory loss can be particularly irritating to the caretaking child. Some sensory loss is predictably correlated with age. Insight can be of great help in this situation. For example, when the parent experiences some hearing loss, the proper response is not necessarily to shout or to lose patience, but, rather, to be willing to repeat as requested, making sure that parent has up-to-date hearing aids, or whatever task-oriented solution is appropriate. Such a response is an insightful action rather than an impulsive reaction. Equally compensatory measures can be applied when other modes of sensory loss occur. While such measures may seem trite, the extent to which the failure to implement them in families with elderly members causes serious problems, necessitates highlighting what appears to be "the obvious."

At the mental or cognitive level, the problems can be more subtle and difficult. Decrements born of, or correlated with, senescence can be more difficult to detect, and they can also be more difficult to diagnose. The practitioner's role in helping the family achieve perspective can be more crucial. The adult child, for example, needs to be aware of the nature of the changes correlated with age, and, perhaps sometimes caused by age. Insight, in fact, can help the adult child become more task oriented. For example, when periods of confusion or short-term memory problems occur, reassurance and mnemonic assistance is required rather than impatience and resignation. Emphasis should be placed on what the parent *can* do instead of what he or she *cannot* do or can do only with untoward difficulty. Proper account should be taken of the fact that there is generally very little, if any, decline in "crystallized intelligence." The skills that one acquires through education and personal experience seem to remain largely intact. Verbal comprehension, numerical reasoning, and inductive reasoning are usually quite stable through the aged years. Understanding the senescence process helps the adult child maintain a balanced perspective and helps preclude the temptation to lose track of the skills the parent retains when some obvious or irritating decrement shows up.

The emotional level is more complex than either of the others, and the assistance of the practitioner in bringing about insight and understanding is often essential. There is the necessary distinction between the acute and the chronic emotional upsets to be dealt with. Without some grasp of the nature of acute, or reversible, behavior disorders, it would be easy, indeed, to make decisions concerning elderly parents that would place their quality of life and their very welfare at considerable risk.

A somewhat simplified but typical scenario might go something like this. The fact is well established that older persons suffer predictable decrements in a number of physical, cognitive, and physiological domains. General vitality and homeostatic constancy is one of them. It takes longer to bounce back from any number of kinds of stress. Sources of stress, moreover, are not lacking. Bereavement, moving, sudden health problems, operations, drug reactions, and other factors can all cause behavior that has a rather sudden onset, and which is aberrant when compared with usual or typical behavior. Statistically, or in terms of incidence, such causes of strange behavior are much more numerous than causes such as some form of organic brain syndrome or generally nonreversible disease. The crucial thing is that the caretaking child understand the concomitants of senescence and the stimulus effect of environmental disequilibration. Instead of becoming unduly alarmed and making decisions for long-term care outside the family group, the individual with the kind of insight based on a general knowledge of senescence and sensitized to the symptoms of reversible symptoms, can look for the probable cause of the aberrant behavior in the life space of the elderly parent. It can often be found. The parent will be his or her old self in short order when the causal agent is identified and set right.

There is always the possibility that one's elderly parent could manifest some form of chronic brain syndrome — perhaps in the severe cases, Pick's or Alzheimer's disease. When the proper clues are present such as gradual and insidious onset and progressively disturbing behavior, the adult child must assess the entire matter from what Keller and Hughston (1981) describe as a "systems" approach. The approach takes into account the entire context in which the behavior occurs with all of its relationships. When the behavior of a parent becomes sufficiently disruptive and persists over a period of time, perhaps the kindest thing for the parent, and certainly for the family, is to place the parent under the care of professionals. This action, difficult as it may be at the time, may be necessary if the family system, basic to the entire network of primary relationships, is to be maintained. Decisions of this kind, however, should be made only after adequate consultation with professionals who have had appropriate experience in such matters.

GENERAL PRINCIPLES

Insight is a quality that enhances most, if not all, relationships; however, to be maximally effective, individuals must be conscious or aware of their insight and must be willing to assume the concomitant or resulting responsibilities; i.e., the burden of the insight.

The principal burden of insight in families involving adult children as caregivers of aged parents, most often falls on one female adult child. The burden is frequently brought into play regarding issues of senescence, generational perspectives, impact of exogenous factors, or conditions that affect the lives of other family members in a major way such as chronic disease or chronic brain syndrome.

Insight is appropriately applied when, under extreme or unduly stressful conditions, objectivity takes precedence over such negative feelings as guilt or misplaced loyalty. The preservation and welfare of self and family should be considered a higher priority than sacrificial behavior toward the aged parent(s).

Behavior born of assuming the burdens of insight can be distinguished from other behavior of a similar nature — selfless or other-oriented behavior — by the presence or absence of perspective. When an individual is conscious of his or her insight or understanding, whether it be of a situation, person, or relationship, and then acts purposefully rather than reacts to some undesirable elements of the situation, perspective is present.

Perspective involves a conscious awareness of the dynamics of a situation or relationship, being able to step aside and view the phenomenon without being caught up in it, then acting in a way as to facilitate the desired outcome. It should be noted, however, that insight can be mutual, but motives and needs may be different. In such an event, outcomes can be highly problematic and confusing to both parties. Such difficulties are best resolved by communication rather than power. Perspective is needed to maintain the necessary balance in such situations.

Finally, the burden of insight is, or tends to be, a form of useful altruism tempered with understanding, perspective and judgement. When one or all parties to a conflicted situation act with insight, things get better. Conversely, when either insight is not present or the key individuals do not assume the burden of responsibility for congruent behavior, things get worse.

The assumption of insight results in behavior that closely resembles interpersonal competence. The sheer incidence of problem behavior in families involving adult children and their aged parents suggests that insight is often in short supply. The good news is that insight, and assuming the consequent burdens, are skills and qualities that can be developed and improved by almost anyone. This fact alone suggests an extremely important and instrumental role for the professional therapist. The recognition of this truth is, itself, a form of insight.

REFERENCES

Benedict, R. (1938). Continuities and discontinuities in cultural conditioning. *Psychiatry, 1*, 161-167.

Bohm, D. (1981). Insight, knowledge, science, and human values. *Teachers College Record, 82*, 380-402.

Davidson, J. E., & Sternberg, R. J. (1986). What is insight? *Educational Horizens, 64*, 177-179.

Erikson, E. H. (1964). The golden rule in the light of new insight. *Insight and responsibility*. New York: W.W. Norton, 219-243.

Freud, A. (1981). Insight: Its presence and absence as a factor in normal development. *Psychoanalytic Study of the Child, 36*, 241-249.

Keller, F. K., & Hughston, G. A. (1981). *Counseling the elderly*. New York: Harper and Row.

Lewis, A. M., & Lewis, S. K. (1986). Intergenerational conflict: Consideration for clergy. *Pastoral Psychology, 35*(1), 46-49.

Waller, W., & Hill, R. (1951). *The family*. New York: The Dryden Press.

Solution Focused Psychotherapy with Families Caring for an Alzheimer's Patient

Marilyn J. Bonjean

SUMMARY. Alzheimer's disease, a progressive and global impairment of the brain, is the fourth leading cause of death in the elderly. Caring for an Alzheimer's patient impacts upon the patient's family as communication patterns, roles, relationships, and family structure change to accommodate care. The model of psychotherapy proposed in this chapter is based upon a solution focused systemic strategic theory of family therapy with families of Alzheimer's patients. Treating the family unit can guide caregivers to a plan of care appropriate for the family developmental and relationship context and flexible enough to allow the needs of all members to be considered.

Alzheimer's disease, a progressive and global impairment of the brain, is the fourth leading cause of death in the elderly, claiming 120,000 lives each year. Estimates place the incidence at about three million afflicted persons, indicating the involvement of approximately 12 million family members (Mace and Rabins, 1981). Alzheimer's disease is characterized by abnormal brain structures of unknown causes: senile plaques, neurofibrillary tangles and granuovascullar structures (Gurland et al., 1980). It follows a progressive course of gradual decline in memory and judgment and is a terminal illness.

Caring for an Alzheimer's disease patient has an impact upon the patient's whole family and especially upon the primary caregiver. Leisure time, privacy, social contacts, physical well being and

Marilyn J. Bonjean, EdD, is Director of Social Services, Marian Catholic Home, and Research Associate, Brief Family Therapy Center, Milwaukee, WI.

emotional stability are all affected (Rabins et al., 1982; Goldman and Luchins, 1984; Tusink and Mahler, 1984; George and Gwyther, 1986; Zarit et al., 1986). Memory disturbance is the most problematic behavior for caregivers of elderly persons. The correlation between cognitive incapacity and burden is significant and suggests that the patient's forgetfulness leads the caregiver to a constant stressful need to compensate for decreasing judgment (Poulshock and Deimling, 1984). Clearly those caring for an Alzheimer's patient are themselves at risk for mental and physical health problems. Mental health concerns are those most commonly reported by family caregivers (George and Gwyther, 1986). Caregivers fear death themselves as they observe the approaching death of the care receiver, are plagued by anxiety resulting from social isolation, and struggle with establishing a purposeful personal life (Levine et al., 1984).

Much of the research related to caregiving has focused upon primary caregivers for Alzheimer's patients since the care situation hinges upon their well being and they are most at risk for developing physical and psychological stress symptoms. A review of this literature indicates that the primary caregiver is at least twice as likely to be a woman as a man. A male care receiver is most often cared for by his wife and a female care receiver by her daughter or daughter-in-law. Women providing care are 65 or older if caring for a spouse or mid to late fifties if caring for a parent (Brody, 1985). When husbands provide care for their wives, Stone et al. (1986) found them to be the oldest group of caregivers putting in the most extra hours in caregiving activities. More than one-half provided care with no informal support or paid assistance.

INDIVIDUAL THERAPY
FOR THE PRIMARY CAREGIVER

Various authors have emphasized the importance of individual psychotherapy for the primary caregiver. Groves et al. (1984) reported that spouses receiving psychotherapy showed symptomatic relief and that in some cases there was a successful resolution of a focal conflict with the demented relative. Zarit and Zarit (1982) found that caregivers requested help at times of such great stress that they benefited from the immediate relief of individual sessions more than joining a support group. Toseland et al. (1984) and Ware and Carper (1982) have also suggested benefits from individual therapy.

FAMILY THERAPY FOR CAREGIVERS

Little attention has been drawn to the family system as it responds to the patient's decline. Secondary caregivers often assist the primary caregiver but do not usually live with the demented person. Those who are geographically close have concerns about their part in the direct caregiving arrangements (George, 1986) and those farther away are concerned about receiving information regarding the evolving care situation and providing emotional support for the primary carer. They will all experience changes in communication patterns, role relationships, family structure (Boss, 1984), grieve the loss of their relative and wonder about the potential for genetic inheritance. Previous conflicts may be reawakened and played out in the context of care provision.

The model proposed in this chapter is based upon the author's clinical experience utilizing a solution focused systemic strategic theory of family therapy (de Shazer, 1985) with families of Alzheimer's patients. It proposes that Alzheimer's patients are members of a family interactional system spanning several generations which influence the implementation of an effective care plan for the patient. Family therapy can generate support from family and friends which appears to mediate much of the stress of caregiving. The usefulness of family meetings has been described (Zarit and Zarit, 1982) and Lezak (1978) and Henry, Knippa, and Golden (1985) have stressed the need for family therapy as part of an intervention plan.

Beginning Therapy

The first family contact often comes from a stressed primary caregiver or a secondary caregiver worried about the caretaking situation. The therapist will need to determine who is part of this family and therefore needs to be included in the therapy in some manner.

Each family member will have a unique view of the caretaking situation, of the illness itself, and past relationship with the patient as well as other family members. Understanding how each family member thinks will allow the therapist to build rapport and form a realistic basis for the problem solving process. An interest in and validation of the views and contributions of all members will put them at ease and allow for creation of a care plan which has broad family support.

Patients in the early stages of the illness can often be included in some of the sessions which allows for discussion of their preferences in developing a care plan and often relieves the family of guilt about decisions. For example, Mrs. Wilson called for an appointment because she needed to make a decision about continuing to live in a large country home or moving to a smaller home in the city which would be easier to maintain and closer to services for her husband who was in the early stages of Alzheimer's disease. Her son and daughter tried to offer her advice but had some ambivalent feelings about selling the family home. Mrs. Wilson had said little to her husband about this decision because she felt it would make him too anxious. When the patient was included in sessions with his family, he was able to be very realistic about his inability to continue the home maintenance he had previously performed and to share his feelings of being overwhelmed by the yard work. He was also able to discuss his fears about selling the house because he had never done this before and knew his memory problem would make it difficult. As the family discussed this issue, they were able to decide to sell the house and the role each would take in the sale. Mrs. Wilson was relieved of the burden of sole decision making and guilt over future problems associated with the move. Mr. Wilson felt his views counted and that he could contribute to the family. An open discussion of this issue allowed the children to be more comfortable discussing their father's illness and so diminished the isolation many patients and caregivers feel when others try to overly protect them.

Giving Information

The therapist will need to determine whether the recommended physical and psychological evaluation for mental impairment has been conducted. Zarit et al. (1985) provide an explanation of psychological testing and the Alzheimer's diagnosis while medical evaluation is thoroughly discussed by Katzman (1986) and in the National Institute on Aging Report (1980). This is very important because many treatable conditions may include some degree of memory disturbance. Even though the diagnosis may have been carefully made and explained to the family, the need for accurate information from the therapist will be essential throughout the course of therapy. Each family member will have a personal timetable for absorbing the diagnosis and adjusting to the patient's disabilities. This is often difficult for secondary caregivers when the patient looks quite normal and displays little abnormal behavior in social situations or the primary caregiver expertly compensates for the patient. Rather than a denial of reality to be overcome, this is either a lack of information or a functional stress regulation. If the therapist can continue to give information, family members will absorb it as they are able.

Treatment Issues

Caregiving families will bring a variety of issues to treatment. As the patient's memory and judgment fail, depression, paranoia, wandering, incontinence, constant repetition, belligerence, and assaultive behavior can mentally and physically exhaust caregivers. The progressive losses and restructuring of family roles can produce strong, confusing emotional responses. A puzzling mixture of grief, guilt, anger, embarrassment and love, satisfaction, patience, and perseverance need to be normalized.

Relationships between family members can range along a continuum from very positive to extremely dysfunctional. Any care decisions must be made with realistic consideration for each individual's and family's history, qualitative relationships, life stage and coping capacity. For example, a care plan for a family in which the primary caregiver is a mid-life daughter and single parent, caring for a widowed mother who has been physically abusive must be very different from the plan of a family in which the primary care-giver is an elderly, physically healthy spouse assisted by several committed children and grandchildren.

Families may enter therapy at any time during the course of the illness from prediagnosis questioning, to accepting the diagnosis, during the years of extended care, at the terminal stage or while mourning the patient's death. Families at each phase will bring unique issues and need to organize differently to meet the challenges of care.

Since Alzheimer's disease has a gradual onset, the patient may be symptomatic for several years before the failure of memory and judgment become significant to other family members. Often a marker event occurs which forces others to notice a difference too great to be ignored; the homemaker who can no longer make coffee, the accountant who cannot write a check or the retired cab driver who forgets the way home. The realization of a significant difference leads the family on a search for answers — a diagnosis. The diagnostic protocol for probable Alzheimer's disease has become much more precise but this information has not reached every physician. Some families still have many problems obtaining a diagnosis other than old age, senility, or organic brain syndrome. These families will have great difficulty in adjustment since the giving of a diagnostic label helps the family to symbolize what is happening to them, to educate themselves and others, project the course of the illness and plan for care. Obtaining a diagnosis allows for the necessary grieving of the pre-illness family identity and acceptance of a permanent change.

After the diagnostic process is completed, the family will move through a transition from pulling together during the crisis of diagnosis to an organization which can sustain years of chronic care. A balance must be struck between appropriate care for the patient and the individual development of each family member.

Since the duration of this illness is difficult to predict, the care-taking task has an open ended nature which requires the family to create a careful balance between its energy and development and new caretaking tasks. Continuous adaptation will make "normal life" routines difficult to maintain since often just as the family unit feels competent in managing certain behaviors the patient changes.

The provision of care for a member will create an inward family focus which emphasizes interior family process. If the illness occurs when the family unit is normally engaged in greater differentiation or disengagement, as when launching adolescents, the opposing forces will make balancing autonomy for each member with the pull of mutual dependence a tremendous challenge. If the illness occurs when the family unit is normally engaged in focusing upon its own processes such as the birth of children, the illness will intensify the already existing interior forces and make moving toward individuation difficult (Combrinck-Graham, 1985). Clear self-expectations must be formulated for each family member so that the well being of the entire family unit is not sacrificed to the care of one person.

Most families will need help from community resources at some time during their caretaking career. However many wait to utilize such assistance until the caregivers are exhausted or the situation is in jeopardy. Stone et al. (1986) found only ten percent of caregivers using community resources. In a recent survey of 289 caregivers (Chenoweth and Spencer, 1986), none reported being given information about home services when the diagnosis and care plan were discussed with the physician. The therapist must decide when a referral is needed, be familiar with quality resources, and help the family accept outside help. Adult day care, home health care, in-home respite, home delivered meals and special transportation services could be useful in easing the burden for the primary caregiver. Contributions of time or financial support from the family can give secondary caregivers an important opportunity to enhance the quality of life for patient and primary caregiver. Legal and financial planning will be important so that providing care does not impoverish the family (Gilfix, 1984).

As the chronic phase draws to a close and the patient becomes imminently terminal, another transition occurs which requires letting go of the structure which has supported care for so long so that the patient can die with peace and dignity. This transition will require the family unit to share strong emotions of grief and mourning.

The terminal phase of the illness brings the need to participate in making terminal care preferences clear to the medical team, clarification of the appropriate use of a nursing home, accepting ambivalent feelings of grief and relief and beginning to plan for a future without the patient.

Solution Focused Intervention

The family will begin treatment focused upon the patient as the problem. As treatment progresses, the therapist will create a shift of focus to the family as a whole and how they will adapt to dependence, deterioration and loss while protecting the individual development of each member. As family members describe the way in which the illness is affecting them, the problem and solution can be redefined in family terms. Although painful and frightening, the illness provides at least an opportunity for responsible behavior and at best increased family solidarity.

Solution focused therapy assumes that clients have the resources for problem solving and that the goal of therapy is to guide them in this process (de Shazer, 1982, 1985). The therapist creates a focus on client strengths and solutions through sequences of questions carefully formulated to evoke different thoughts, feelings, perceptions and behaviors about complaints (Lipchik, 1988). The early treatment process centers around promoting a description of any exceptions to the problem. An exception is what is happening when the problem does not occur or is variable in intensity.

Descriptions of the complaint will have some variation since there is always asynchronicity in any pattern under consideration. The therapist in this model chooses a focus on the positive elements of the partial and changing fit between elements of a behavior pattern. Focus on the problem at the initiation of therapy maintains and expands this framework while a solution focus encourages the family to observe what they are doing right and to increase those behaviors. The therapist highlights the smallest difference between the solution framework and that of the complaint through obtaining thorough descriptions of exceptions, recent changes or if necessary imagined possible solutions. For example, Mrs. Williams' daughter called for an appointment because she was concerned about her mother's depressed feelings and fluctuating hypertension. Mrs. Williams, her daughter, and son attended the first session. Her husband who was in the very late stages of Alzheimer's disease and required complete care remained at home. A thorough medical history of the husband had been forwarded to the therapist before the session. The daughter begins by describing why the family had come:

Daughter: We are very concerned about Mother and wanted to come for consultation because we're really afraid she'll have a stroke. She seems so down all the time and her blood pressure is out of control.

Son: Yes, Mom is really wearing out taking care of Dad but she won't hear of any help.

Therapist: Mrs. Williams, obviously your children are very concerned for you. You are under a doctor's care for your hypertension. What does she say about your blood pressure?

The therapist asks about her medical treatment because this is part of an exception to illness or something the client is doing right to help herself and should be noted. Later it can be reflected as one method of self-care she already has in place.

Mrs. Williams: She says that my medication needs some adjustment so I've been changing the time when I take some of my pills. I brought them in this bag like you asked. She says my blood pressure problem is mainly stress.

The therapist takes the bag so that later during the intervention break the medication can be noted for future review and perhaps discussion with the physician. Medication interaction could play a part in her emotional reactions.

Therapist: So you have been consulting with a physician regularly to try to stay healthy. Your children say they are also concerned about your feeling down a lot. Are there any times when you feel just a little bit better.

Here instead of exploring the depression further from the vantage point of the problem, the therapist will explore exceptions and focus on possible pieces of the solution.

Mrs. Williams: You know it is funny. I feel more down now than I did when my sister was dying.

Daughter: Mom, you can't mean that. I thought you were so hurt by Aunt Betty's death and you were dragging yourself to the hospital for weeks. I've been telling you you've got to stop thinking about her all the time.

Therapist: Mrs. Williams, how do you account for feeling better then?

Mrs. Williams: I don't know. I was going back and forth a lot then and I had an attendant and the children caring for my husband. I do it myself now, of course. I miss Betty but I really felt less down. The children were so good to me then, so supportive.

At this point the therapist has information about a difference between the past and present depression level of Mrs. Williams. The therapist can continue to explore with the family hypotheses about this positive difference. Is it the respite of being away from her husband, the increased family solidarity during crisis, the use of community resources, the need to be allowed a period of grieving? All those possibilities and more can be explored through questioning the family. As the behaviors and attitudes of each are explored, pieces of a solution framework will become evident so that the family can arrive at a care plan which respects the needs of each and provides appropriate care for the patient.

Homework Assignments

At the end of each session the therapist will develop a homework assignment which has been carefully tailored to fit the language and world view of each family member. The homework begins with a "compliment" portion which focuses on the strengths of family members and what they are doing right. Then a request is added for each to do, think about or observe something. For example, at the conclusion of the session with the Williams family excerpted in the preceding the following homework assignment might be given: (Compliment) I am very impressed with the concern each of you has for the others in your family and your willingness to seek consultation when it seemed needed. Your children's concern for you shows me that you, Mrs. Williams, and your husband did a lot of things right as their parents. Part of your depression is, of course, a normal response to your sister's death and you intuitively know you must not try to get over that too fast. You must honor your grief and your children need to support your doing that. (Exception) However, you have discovered that when you were out of the house more, even if visiting your dying sister, you still felt better in a way. It seems that being away from your husband for periods of time is helpful. Of course, it is difficult to ask for help and yet is essential if you are to stay well enough to continue to care for him. (Task) Between now and the next time we meet I would like all of you to think about how you will be able to get more time for yourself, Mrs. Williams.

Each subsequent session will begin with an examination of how the task was carried out. It could be completed as requested, modified, or not completed which is information useful to the therapist in designing future tasks. The focus on exceptions to the problem will continue so that the client moves toward an emphasis on thoughts, feelings, and behaviors outside of the complaint frame.

Blocking Overly Rapid Solution

Under stress family members will utilize old patterns of problem solving which may not be useful. An expedient solution which places an unrealistic burden upon one member or does not take note of past family relationships is temporary at best and at worst creates another patient. The therapist will need to block too rapid attempts at solution for the sake of tension reduction and encourage planning which is very realistic and commitments which are made only after thoughtful dialogue within the family.

Diffusing Old Battles

For some families, the stress of caring for a mentally impaired member will reawaken unresolved resentments, anger or even hatred. These feelings can block the family from reaching consensus on a plan of care. The family therapist in this model will acknowledge the presence of such relationships as part of the interactional system but will not focus attention on those issues. The therapist will attend to this history only as it relates to the family's ability to care for a member and develop a plan realistically based upon the family context. Understanding how the family unit has coped with crisis and conflict will help the therapist discover any behaviors which have been successful for this family. Families may have coped with progressive, chronic illness and death or may have experienced acute, nonfatal illnesses. Behaviors which were useful in acute situations can be adapted to be useful in situations of extended care for chronic illness.

Termination

As family therapy reaches termination, the therapist can help family members prepare for the future by predicting future cycles of ambiguity. Since Alzheimer's disease is a progressive illness, the condition of the patient will continue to change and the family must adjust accordingly. The family as a unit will also change over time and may find it helpful to generate contingency plans with the therapist which take these predictable developments into consideration. Family members can be prepared by the therapist to recognize cycles of ambiguity; confusion about changes in the patient, gathering information, trying new resources or approaches, and incorporating into family functioning behaviors appropriate to managing change.

CONCLUSION

Although the terminal illness of a member may stress the family unit to its capacity, it also provides an opportunity for members to behave responsibly toward each other so that this life event does not generate problems for future generations. Treating the family unit allows the therapist to guide caregivers to a plan of care which is appropriate for the family developmental and relationship context and is flexible enough to allow for the needs of all members to be considered. Although they may always have some resentments, guilt or ambivalent feelings, family members can cooperate in managing problems and diffusing tension to preserve the health of the family system.

REFERENCES

Brody, E.M. (1985). Parent care as a normative family stress. *The Gerontologist*, 25, 19-29.

Chenoweth, B. and Spencer, B. (1986). Dementia: The experience of family caregivers. *The Gerontologist*, 26, 267-272.

Combrinck-Graham, L. (1985). A developmental model for family systems. *Family Systems*, 24, 139-150.

de Shazer, S. (1985). *Keys to solution in brief therapy*. New York: W.W. Norton, Inc.

_____. (1982). *Pattern of brief family therapy*. New York: The Guilford Press.

George, L. (1986). Caregiver burden: Conflict between norms of reciprocity and solidarity. In K. Pillemer and R. Wolf (eds.) *Elder abuse – conflict in the family*. Dover, Mass: Auburn House Publishing Company.

George, L.K. and Gwyther, L.P. (1986). Caregiver well-being a multidimensional examination of family caregivers of demented adults. *The Gerontologist*, 26, 253-259.

Gilfix, M. (1984). Legal strategies for patient and family. *Generations*, 9 (Winter), 46-48.

Goldman, L.S. and Luchins, D.J. (1984). Depression in the spouses of demented patients. *American Journal of Psychiatry*, 141, 1467-1468.

Groves, L., Lazarus, L.W., Newton, N., Frankel, R., Gutmann, D.L. and Ripeckyj, A. (1984). Brief psychotherapy with spouses of patients with Alzheimer's disease: Relief of the psychological burden. In L.W. Lazarus (ed.) *Clinical approaches to psychotherapy with elderly*. Washington, D.C.: American Psychiatric Press.

Gurland, B., Dean, L., Craw, P. and Golden, R. (1980). The epidemiology of depression and delirium in the elderly: The use of multiple indicators of these conditions. In J.O. Cole and J.E. Barret (eds.) *Psychopathology in the aged*. New York: Raven Press.

Henry, P., Knippa, J. and Golden, C. (1985). A systems model for therapy with brain-injured adults and their families. *Family Systems Medicine*, 3, 427-439.

Katzman, R. (1986). Alzheimer's disease. *New England Journal of Medicine*, 314, 964-973.

Levine, N.D., Gendron, C.E., Dastoor, D.P., Poitras, L.R., Sirota, S.E., Barza, S.L. and Davis, J.C. (1984). Existential issues in management of the demented elderly patient. *American Journal of Psychotherapy*, 38, 215-223.

Lezak, M. (1978). Living with the characterologically altered brain injured patient. *The Journal of Clinical Psychiatry*, 39, 592-598.

Lipchik, E. (1988). Purposeful interviewing for beginning the solution-focused interview. In E. Lipchik (ed.) *Interviewing*. Rockville, Md.: Aspen Publishers.

Mace, N.L. and Rabins, P.V. (1981). *The 36-hour day a family guide to caring for people with Alzheimer's disease, related dementing illness and memory loss in late life*. Baltimore: John's Hopkins University.

National Institute on Aging Task Force. (1980). Senility reconsidered: Treatment possibilities for mental impairment in the elderly. *Journal of American Medical Association*, 244, 259-263.

Poulshock, S.W. and Deimling, G.T. (1984). Families caring for elders in residence: Issues in measurement of burden. *Journal of Gerontology*, 39, 230-239.

Rabins, P.V., Mace, N.L. and Lucas, M.J. (1982). The impact of dementia on the family. *Journal of the American Medical Association*, 248, 333-335.

Stone, R., Cafferata, G.L. and Sangl, J. (1986). *Caregivers of the frail elderly: A national profile*. National Center for Health Services Research, Publications and Information Branch, Rockville, Md.

Toseland, R.W., Denico, A. and Owen, M.L. (1984). Alzheimer's disease and related disorders: Assessment and intervention. *Health and Social Work*, 9, 212-226.

Tuesink, J. and Mahler, S. (1984). Helping families cope with Alzheimer's disease. *Hospital and Community Psychiatry*, 35, 152-156.

Ware, L. and Carper, M. (1982). Living with Alzheimer's disease patients: Family stresses and coping mechanisms. *Psychotherapy: Theory, Research, and Practice*, 19 (Winter), 472-481.

Zarit, S.H., Todd, P.A. and Zarit, J.M. (1986). Subjective burden of husband and wife caregivers: A longitudinal study. *The Gerontologist*, 26, 260-266.

Zarit, S.H., Orr, N.K. and Zarit, J.M. (1985). *The hidden victims of Alzheimer's disease families under stress*. New York: University Press.

Zarit, S.H. and Zarit, J.M. (1982). Families under stress: Interventions for caregivers of senile dementia patients. *Psychotherapy: Theory, Research, and Practice*, 19, 461-471.

Retirement
and the Contemporary Family

Neil Gerard McCluskey

SUMMARY. Profound changes in the nation's demographic patterns have transformed life for contemporary Americans. People 65 years of age and over now comprise a much larger segment of the population. They are both living longer and living more healthily. An additional 27 years has been added to the life span of the child of 1985 as compared to a child born in 1900, so that the problems and solutions of today will not be final but must continue to command the attention of the public. These changes are affecting family life. The meaning of retirement has changed. The timetable for retirement is a new one. The needs of the retiring and retirement population have changed. The article discusses new ways of confronting these needs. Eldercare is seriously affecting the workplace. The seeming dilemma, faced especially by female employees, in choosing between working at a career and providing home care for a vulnerable relative, may have a resolution. More outside help is available to the family than at any earlier period so that helping an aging relative no longer has to mean dedicating one's entire life to providing eldercare. The ideal still is to maintain independent living for both the active and frail elderly as long as practically possible. Family and friends of the frail elderly no longer have to carry the burden alone. A spectrum of in-home services is available to families across the land.

CHARACTERISTICS OF TODAY'S ELDERLY

Profound changes in the nation's demographic pattern have heralded for most people the prospect of a longer life than was dreamed of by prior generations. Like any number of other Western soci-

Neil Gerard McCluskey, PhD, is Senior Consultant, R.A.I. Division, Hearst Business Publications, 919 3rd Avenue, New York, NY 10022.

eties, the United States is only slowly and haphazardly adjusting to this reality. Science and medicine have extended life expectancy, but society is only beginning to adjust to the implications of a longer life — as if mankind could not believe such a good thing were truly taking place. The response is reactive. Most people are not given to solid planning.

Older people now comprise a larger component of the total population, and their absolute and relative numbers will continue to increase for the remainder of this century and into the next. More Americans are living longer, and older Americans are living to a more advanced age. Today some 30 million (12%) of all Americans are 65 or over — nearly one in eight. Of these, 11.5 million are men and 17 million are women, a ratio of 100 to 147. The sex ratio decreases with age, ranging from 100 to 122 for the 65-59 group to a low of 100 to 251 for those 85 and older. Projections are that the number of the 65-plus group will be 35 million in the year 2000 and 40 million in 2010. The growth will slow somewhat in the 1990s, reflecting the lower birth rate during the years of the Great Depression. Between 2010 and 2030, the "Baby Boom" of the post-World War II years will become the "Gray Explosion." This 20-year period (only 32 years away) is expected to see the most rapid increase of seniors in our history with the result that by 2030 there will be *65 million* 65-year-olds and older. They are expected to make up 21.2% of the population. This total represents two and one-half times their number in 1980.

In 1985, the 65-74 age group of 17 million was 8 times larger than in 1900, the 75-84 group of 8.8 million was 11 times larger, and the 85-plus group of 2.7 million was 22 times larger. A child born in 1900 could expect to live just under 48 years. A child born in 1985 can expect to live to 74.7 years, an addition of 27 years.

Geriatricians have observed that today's 60-year-olds resemble 40-year-olds of a century ago "in terms of the aging process as evidenced by muscular agility and strength, skin turgor, and other indices of youthfulness vs. senescence" (Stevenson, 1979).

The average American man or woman at 65 is vigorous, alert, and independent. He or she pursues an active, productive, and meaningful life, a living refutation of the negative stereotypes of old age that still pervade our culture. It is factual that 95% of the 65-

plus population form a regular part of the everyday world, and that only 5% are confined to nursing homes. Some 91% of the 75-and-over population remain active in the day-to-day world and only 9% are in nursing homes.

Hence, the question can be raised as to whether the word "senior" should be more appropriately reserved for people who have passed their 75th year. More and more, the terms "young old" for those under 75 and "old old" for those who have passed that milestone are coming into the terminology. These new terms seem much more accurate for characterizing older individuals.

With all these assuring positive things said, however, there is another side to the aging pattern. In general, men and women past 65 do visit doctors more often, take more medication, and spend more time in hospitals than do younger people. Of the 65-plus group, three-quarters suffer at least one chronic disease and nearly one-half have some limitation upon daily activities. On the other hand, it is also factual that many of the changes in later life have little or nothing to do with aging. Most of the malfunctioning in the bodily systems of the elderly can be traced to either hereditary weakness, environmental harm, or self-inflicted damage.

PREPARING FOR CHANGE

Only in recent years have the problems and needs of the aging population commanded substantial public attention. Only in recent years has the nation begun to regard its elderly not simply as consumers of services but to respect them as potential providers of services. Both the elderly themselves and their adult children anticipate the years past 60 as the worst part of adult life — a period of possible loneliness, inactivity and poor health. Beyond doubt, the main reason for this situation is the lack of proper planning or preparation for what we have traditionally called the "retirement years" but which some writers prefer to call the "late adult years." The two terms are no longer synonymous.

Given the combination of increased longevity and improved health of today's older population, adult children and families generally will not have to meet the responsibility of caring for their elderly as soon as preceding generations did. Nor will they be giving the same kind of care. For discussion purposes, we can divide the span of care into two separate but sometimes overlapping phases: the independent years, and the dependent years, with the 75-80 year period serving as a very arbitrary divider.

Retirement at any age is usually a traumatic or at the least, a dramatic, experience. A good first step in psychological preparation would be to banish the word "retirement" from the language. Failing that, conscious effort should be made to endow the term with a more positive meaning so that it more accurately reflects the social reality.

Since retirement planning came into being, the emphasis has generally been on retirement as a *terminal* event after a lifetime of work. At times it was welcomed as a surcease from toil or accepted as an earned reward. Where persons looking at retirement experienced dread, it was mainly because of their social conditioning. They connected retirement with such stereotypes as being "at the end of the line," "on the shelf," "over the hill," or "put out to pasture." These cliches no longer fit today's men and women who bring healthy bodies and sound minds to their 62nd or 65th or 70th or 75th birthdays. They may leave full-time employment, but they are unlike the retirees of earlier generations.

For them, emphasis now is on continuity of activity, the life-span nature of the process—not a retirement *from* but a retirement *to* something new but normal. In response to this new understanding, different conceptual models have been advanced to explain the sequence of events in a mature person's life that call for plans and decisions.

In the literature, we now find such terms as "stages," "seasons," "passages," and "transitions" (Levinson, 1978; Sheehy, 1976; and others). This writer prefers "transfer point in life" as the most accurate concept of retirement, "point" for the event and "transfer" for the implication of dynamic change. Transfer point is where an adult person changes from one vehicle or track to another, where he or she transfers skills and talents from one set of tasks to another, where he or she can shift priorities and change the tempo of activity.

Likewise, the retirement event itself can be construed as the document of transfer which admits a person to a new vehicle or track.

Transfer applies to the area of finance in the choice of pension options or new income-generating investments. Transfer also is involved in the realignment of medical and hospital support through enrollment in group plans or special insurance. Transfer can be applicable to decisions regarding change of residence and lifestyle. Transfer covers the development of new activities, interests and goals. In sum, the transfer is a transition into a new phase of mature adult life with its own special expectancies, tasks and challenges.

In helping prepare an elderly parent or relative for assuming the new role, whatever one chooses to call it, the family can play a significant part. The 65- or 70-year-old parent should be encouraged to plan ahead for the kind of active life commensurate with his or her physical and mental strength, psychological needs and ambitions. However, adult children should not attempt to reverse the parent-child relationship. Functioning as friend and confidant who respects and trusts an older friend, adult children should be encouraging and supportive. In this way, they can smooth the transition and help their elder loved ones to develop new lifestyles. With family sharing in the preparation, unpleasant surprises can be avoided.

So the day finally arrives when dad or mom collects the final pay check from full-time employment. He or she no longer has an office or work station to go to every weekday morning at 8:00. The delight of unbounded leisure fades rather quickly. More than the diminished income (ordinarily a drop of 50%), retirees initially miss the regular routine of work. This is a natural reaction, for we all tend to define ourselves by what we do. The second question asked when strangers meet is usually, "What do you do?"

Family can again be most helpful here. Newly retired parents can be encouraged to strike out in new directions of activity or interest. They can be counseled and assisted to become occupied in new or renewed pursuits, part-time work, new skills or hobbies, travel, education, volunteer and charitable activities, and many other meaningful enterprises.

During the active period before the inevitable slowdown, adult children can help their parents clarify the financial base upon which they must live. To conserve or increase financial resources, they can help arrange for the expert help of an estate planner. Working with the planner and the elder parent, they can remove much of the concern over finances that is a principal source of stress for the elderly. They can assist in helping to assure income stability, adequate health and hospital insurance, and comfortable housing.

TIME FOR THE CAREGIVER

Each year past age 75, the likelihood of the need for more systematic intervention by an outside agent or agency increases. There is almost an inevitable need for at least close surveillance over the lives of those beyond 85. And this is the segment of the elderly population that is expanding most rapidly. Between 1960 and 1980, this age group increased by 165%. These "oldest old" will total five million by the end of the century. There are few, if any, historical precedents to measure the long-term consequences this radical change will have on family life and in the workplace.

A decade ago, it was assumed in the literature that the surviving elderly were largely abandoned by their families to live in lonely isolation or to be dispatched to a nursing home. More recent research has shown the situation to be considerably different.

In 1985, an estimated 1.4 million elderly Americans did live in nursing homes. However, another 5.2 million lived in the community with some level of disability that left them in need of help with day-to-day tasks. Now we know that the majority of the elderly live at home but do require the level of help that family members can usually give, supplemented by professional services. Of those 85-years-of-age and older, most are widows and only 22%, approximately one in five, live in homes for the elderly. It is the members of this age group who are most likely to be in need of care.

Families, then, not government or agency programs, provide the bulk of personal care which allows these older people to remain in the community. In fact, research has indicated that families provide 80 to 90% of this care. In 1982, there were 7.6 million informal caregivers providing unpaid assistance to 4.3 million elderly who needed assistance with everyday activities.

A 1986 survey of caregivers conducted by Retirement Advisors, Inc. (RAI), a national leader in the retirement planning field, found that 30% of a national sample of employees aged 50-64 were providing some degree of care for an elder, while an additional 10%

anticipated the need in the near future. One third of the care-recipients were women and another third were husband-wife teams. Other studies indicate substantially the same findings (Travelers, 1985; New York Business Group on Health, 1986; National Center for Health Services Research, 1986).

The RAI survey indicates that the vast majority of caregivers are women, either female spouses or middle-aged daughters. A caregiver's average age is 57.3 years; one-quarter are aged 65-74; and 10% are 75 years and over. Three out of four caregivers live with the care receiver. About one-fourth of the daughters and other female caregivers have competing family obligations. The majority of caregivers provide assistance seven days a week, with an average of four hours of service daily or a weekly total of 28 hours.

Indications now are that women will spend more years caring for older family members than they do caring for their own children. Yet, increasingly, these women today are working beyond their fifties, and, consequently, are not at home to care for elderly relatives. Labor statisticians tell us that by 1990, some 70% of women between 35 and 44 are expected to be in the labor force. For women 45 to 54, that percentage will be 61 as compared to 35% in the early 1950s. This change will significantly effect the pool of caregivers who have traditionally cared for the infirm elderly in their homes.

IMPACT OF CAREGIVING ON THE WORKPLACE

For anyone employed full-time, caregiving can translate into reduced on-the-job effectiveness, chronic tardiness, unplanned absenteeism, excessive telephone interruptions, and overall stress. The executive can cushion this impact somewhat by reason of his or her more flexible schedule and staff support. For the average employee without such resources, however, caregiver demands mean problems at work as well as impaired ability to handle outside responsibilities.

Compounding the situation is the fact that the average employee and employer are both uninformed and inexperienced with the American system of support for the aged. Whether in person or by telephone, it is a common experience to meet confusion, frustration, and even degradation when attempting to access the system. A vast array of support programs for the elderly is available today and their number will continue to increase. However, obtaining access is difficult since admission and service delivery systems span a confusing maze of federal, state and local organizations and agencies.

What kinds of care are given? The RAI and other studies have found that many caregivers are responsible for an elder's transportation, bathing and personal care, shopping, cooking, and desk work. Though some of these chores can be taken care of before or after work hours, much of this work is likely to be on company time because the hours of government, medical and professional offices normally are the same as those of the corporate world.

The growing number of caregivers in the workforce is increasingly attracting the attention of employers, social service agencies, healthcare providers, women's organizations, and the major levels of government. The need to come to terms with this issue is obvious. The problem will only grow more urgent in the years immediately ahead. In fact, it is hard to quarrel with the assertion that eldercare will be one of the critical social issues for the remainder of the twentieth century. The elderly population has doubled since 1960 and, by 2030, will do so again. Accordingly, the need for caregivers will also double, a need that will inevitably have profound repercussions on several million more American homes. Though we have discussed, in this section, the impact of eldercare upon the workplace, the impact is being felt equally, if not more, upon the American family. More and more working persons, usually women, will have to face the dilemma of choosing between the continuation of a career or the caring for someone at home. Or will they? Let us see if there is a way out.

MAINTAINING INDEPENDENT LIVING
FOR THE ELDERLY

Most older persons would rather stay in their own homes and communities for as long as possible. A familiar environment with its rich store of memories becomes a kind of extension of the self for the elderly person. Accordingly, a basic rule is that, as long as they are not a threat to their own physical or mental well-being or to that of others, older persons should be encouraged to maintain control over their own lives, preferably in their own homes.

Though the furniture may have become dilapidated and out of style, the neighborhood run down and even a trifle dangerous, mother or dad still find it difficult to make a move to what the whole family may argue is a better place. This is a story that many families can recount. So where do older persons, family members, neighbors and friends turn when someone needs assistance to remain in their homes and communities? This same question is asked by family members who live at a distance, worried because mother or father seem to be having great difficulty in coping with every day living functions around their home, and no one in the family is there to help.

Are adult children the only option? Or is there an alternative to their becoming the direct care providers? In some cases adult children might be able to become the principal caregivers, and it could be an ideal solution. However, in most instances, the immediate family situation makes this arrangement impossible or at least highly impractical on a long-term basis.

In every community, resources are now available to help people care for a frail or dependent relative or friend. Unfortunately, it may not always be simple to find these resources or easy to take advantage of them; patience and perseverance are needed. Here are some suggestions for getting the help needed.

The local telephone directory will have resources listed under the county or city government blue pages, usually under "Senior Citizens" and "Social Services." Some programs may not exist in small towns or rural areas but may be found on the county or state level.

The first place to which a seeker should turn is the local Area Agency on Aging (AAA). There are 672 Area Agencies on Aging, covering all geographic areas of the nation. These agencies were created as a part of the Older Americans Act, first passed by the Congress in 1965, which describes their basic objective: ". . . to provide for a comprehensive array of community-based, long-term care services adequate to appropriately sustain older people in their communities and in their homes . . . with emphasis on maintaining a continuum of care for the vulnerable elderly." Two-thirds of the

Area Agencies are found within city, county, and other forms of local or regional governments. The other third are private, nonprofit entities that represent multiple communities.

These may instead be titled an Office or Department on Aging or Council on Aging. If one is not listed in the local phone directory, the number and address can be obtained from the National Association of Area Agencies on Aging (NAAAA), Suite 208-West, 600 Maryland Avenue, S.W., Washington, D.C. 20024 (phone 202-484-7520). A Silver Pages Telephone Directory, with a comprehensive listing of services for the elderly, is now available in many communities. Free copies are mailed to all area residents over 60 years old.

Specifically, the Area Agency should serve as the first source of information as to what, how, and where home-care services may be available. Despite a slow beginning and uneven development of the AAA network across the country, more and more recognition is being given to the role of the agencies in assisting elderly persons and their family members to determine what services are needed, how to access them, how to determine whether they are appropriately provided, and what resources are available to support such services.

The range of services is impressive. Some of the in-home supportive services available in communities include:

Chore services	Escort/transportation
Telephone reassurance	Homemaker services
Home visiting	Shopping assistance
Personal care services	Home health aides
Home delivered meals	Home safety checks

If the local Area Agency on Aging does not provide a service themselves, they should be able to put an inquirer in touch with someone who does. In most communities, there is a choice among the nonprofit (voluntary) organizations and the care-provider (proprietary) businesses.

In addition, religious, fraternal, and ethnic groups have a rich tradition of providing care and comfort to the elderly, needy or not. Long before there were state-supported social service programs, groups like the Catholic Sisterhoods and Jewish Landsmen Societies as well as the churches themselves were providing the elderly of their constituencies, and often other elderly, with medical and hospital care, temporary and permanent shelter, and burial. This tradition of voluntary care is still very much alive in the various multi-service programs and institutions in the private sector across the length and breadth of the land.

Then there are also the commercial operations which have had an explosive expansion since the early 1980s. The emergence of a vigorous health care industry in America is hardly to be wondered at, given the tremendous growth of the market, i.e., the aging population. In addition to the traditional health offerings they put on the market for the elderly, these operators have developed and manage a multi-billion dollar retirement housing industry. The financial planning, physical and psychological needs of the elderly population have placed such demands on existing support systems, whether in the private or public sector, that neither the tax-supported programs nor the voluntary sector seems able to keep up with the demand. Hence we see the entrance into the eldercare market of corporate giants, private pension funds, investment bankers, and life insurance companies. No longer is the field dominated by church-related and other nonprofit groups. The trend has been set, and there is no indication that it will soon be reversed. In any event, those who have the most to gain here seem to be the elderly themselves and the families they look to for support.

IN-HOME SERVICES AVAILABLE
TO FAMILIES

In most American communities, there is a range of services designed to assist people to maintain independent living. Let it be remembered that not every community will have them all, but only a few communities will have none. As noted above, in-home services include: home health aide, counseling, homemaking services, home repair, chore services, shopping, friendly visiting, and home-delivered meals. Other extended community services might be offered as well, such as day care, escort, transportation, legal, and information and referral services.

Each of the home-care services comprises an important means for enabling older persons to remain in their own homes. However, the two categories most frequently needed are those of the homemaker and the home health worker. These services maximize an individual's ability to remain in the community, while minimizing the dependency and the loss of human dignity which frequently accompany serious illness and impairment. In addition, the use of these services can prevent or delay institutionalization.

The concern with preventing or delaying institutionalization stems from two sources, the human benefits associated with care in the home, and the rising costs of institutional care.

In closing this paper, let us offer some brief information about Home Health Care and Homemaker Services. It is assumed that these are services delivered by a responsible agency with a professional staff that has well-defined responsibilities for participant assessment, formulation of a care plan, service integration and patient reassessment, as well as an appropriate program of pre-service and in-service training for both professionals and aides.

Home Health Care services, as defined under Medicare, are those provided to an individual under a physician's care by direct arrangement with a home health agency or by others through an arrangement with the agency. These services include nursing, physical therapy, occupational therapy, speech therapy, medical social services, home health aide services, and medical supplies. The same services are available, independent of Medicare, to individuals who may not be under a doctor's care.

Homemaker services are provided by individuals who have had specialized training in both homemaker and home health aide functions. They are able to assume both roles, performing the household management activities associated with homemakers and the personal care activities associated with health aides. They can provide emotional support; assist with food shopping, preparation and eating; help with dressing; do light housekeeping, personal laundry and bed changing; teach home management; provide respite services for family members; and offer special services such as writing of bills and paperwork, and escort services.

BY WAY OF CONCLUSION

The changes within the last four decades that have transformed life for the elderly have, in the process, profoundly affected American family life. The process shows no sign of abating. The meaning of retirement has changed. The timetable is a new one. The needs of the retiring and retired population have changed. There are new ways of meeting these needs. More outside help is available than at any earlier period so that helping an aging relative no longer has to mean giving up one's personal life to provide eldercare. Even so, caregiving almost inevitably brings with it conflict and stress. For those presently involved in this arduous task, it is important to look for partnership, to seek skills and resources from agencies and organizations as a supplement to what the caregiver him- or herself can supply.

It is hoped that the insights and information on eldercare offered here will provide a service to help the family, nuclear or extended, adjust to the new situations of our times.

REFERENCES

Andrus Volunteers (1985). *Who cares? Helpful hints for those who care for a dependent older person at home*. Los Angeles, CA: University of Southern California.

Cadmus, R. R. (1984). *Caring for your aging parents: A concerned complete guide for children of the elderly*. Englewood Cliffs, NJ: Prentice Hall.

Cohen, D., & Eisdorfer, C. (1986). *The loss of self: A family resource for the care of Alzheimer's disease and related disorders*. New York: W. W. Norton and Company.

Horne, J. (1985). *Caregiving: Helping an aging loved one*. Glenview, IL: Scott, Foresman and Company (AARP Books).

McCluskey, N. G., & Borgatta, E. F. (Eds.) (1981). *Aging and retirement: Prospects, planning, and policy*. Beverly Hills, CA: Sage Publications, Inc.

New York City Alzheimer's Resource Center (1985). *Caring: A family guide to managing the Alzheimer's patient at home*. (Developed by F. Tanner with S. Shaw. Available from the New York City Alzheimer's Resource Center, 280 Broadway, Room 214, New York, NY 10007.)

Silverstone, B., & Hyman, H. K. (1982, revised). *You and your aging parent: The modern family's guide to emotional, physical and financial problems*. New York: Pantheon Books.

Thompson, M. K. (1986). *Caring for an elderly relative: A guide to home care.* New York: Prentice Hall.

Tomb, D. A. (1984). *Growing old: A handbook for you and your aging parent.* New York: Viking.

Watt, J., & Calder, A. (1986). *Taking care: A self-help guide for coping with an elderly, chronically ill or disabled relative.* 306 West 25th Street, North Vancouver, British Columbia V7N2G1: International Self-Counsel Press Ltd.

Bereavement and the Elderly:
The Role of the Psychotherapist

Frank R. Williams

SUMMARY. This article explores the subject of dying, death and bereavement, their impact on the elderly person, and the potential for psychotherapeutic intervention. The article discusses the perceptions of the therapist on death and bereavement and on dying and old age and examines the therapeutic process in working with the bereaved.

INTRODUCTION

Beverly Raphael, in her comprehensive work *The Anatomy of Bereavement* (1983), writes:

> Each person must make his way through life encompassing two important facts. If he loves, there will be the great rewards of human intimacy in its broadest sense; and yet when he does so, he becomes vulnerable to the exquisite agony of loss. And one day—he knows not when or how—he will die. (p. 402)

This idea is reiterated by Judith Viorst in the work, *Necessary Losses* (1986):

> I've learned that in the course of one life we leave and are left and let go of much that we love. Losing is the price we pay for living. It is also the source of much of our growth and gain. Making our way from birth to death, we also have to make our

---

Frank R. Williams, ThD, is Family Life Specialist, Cooperative Extension, University of Arizona, Tucson, AZ 85721.

way through the pain of giving up and giving up and giving up
some portion of what we cherish. (pp. 325-326)

As a psychotherapist, there is a constancy that exists in the work
done: helping people work through losses, helping them to do the
necessary grief work. In many ways, it can be said that all therapy
is, in some way, grief work.

In relating to the elderly and their family members, the issues of
loss and bereavement (the state of having lost someone) are ever-
present. There are the functional losses—the impairment of the
body through loss or significant diminishment of vision, hearing,
sexual functioning, or loss of control of other body functions common to many elderly. There are also losses related to role changes
as in retirement when the roles one has carried out, often over a
long period of time, are no longer available. And, for the elderly,
there are the common losses of death—death of friends, of family
and of self.

Everyone who loses someone in death will be bereaved and will
mourn and will experience grief. *Bereavement* is the state of having
experienced the loss of a loved one. A bereaved person is one who
has lost someone. In this article, *grief* refers to the complex painful
effects and the emotional response to loss. *Mourning* is the process
that one goes through in bereavement, including the many and varied rituals associated with the loss. The dying person will mourn
and will experience grief. The family members will do the same.

How one mourns and how one grieves are very different from
one individual to another, depending on the attachment to loved
ones, the cultural background, the person's psychological make-up,
past experiences with loss, and the support system.

Having experienced a loss, then, a person will mourn. That
mourning is a journey of healing that takes time and requires that
certain tasks be completed successfully. It is possible for a person to
accomplish some of the tasks and not others, and, therefore, have
an incomplete bereavement just as one might have incomplete healing from a wound. Mourning will hopefully be concluded with the
bereaved person's emotional healing and on-going adequate life involvement.

The psychotherapist who works with elderly persons or their

families cannot avoid dealing with bereavement. It is a fact of life. This article, therefore, focusses on the psychotherapist's role with the elderly and their family members when confronted with death and the subsequent bereavement.

THE PSYCHOTHERAPIST AND BEREAVEMENT

While it might be said that most therapy is grief therapy, psychotherapists tend to be ill-prepared to deal with bereavement. There are a few therapists who have specialized in bereavement issues, but most psychotherapists are generalists and are not regularly faced with death. In order to work with elderly persons, the psychotherapist must be prepared to work extensively with these issues.

Bereavement presents a special challenge to the psychotherapist. In the face of loss, especially death, the helping person is confronted with his own impotence. He or she faces a sense of helplessness, along with the inevitable pain of being witness to the experience.

Especially important is the psychotherapist's attitude about his or her own mortality, his or her own death. In working with the elderly, death is an ever-present possibility. Death and dying issues put the psychotherapist in touch with the extent to which there is an uncontrollableness of his or her own death. While everyone has some anxiety about dying, the psychotherapist needs to face this anxiety directly lest it become an issue that hinders effectiveness in working with elderly clients.

Psychotherapists working with the elderly are also encouraged to explore their own history of losses, looking at their own process of bereavement and how it has been worked through. If there are unresolved losses, these can be an impediment to a meaningful and helpful intervention. If the therapist's losses have been adequately integrated, these experiences with similar losses can be useful in working with a client. By investigating his or her personal history, the psychotherapist can explore what were positive resources in bereavement and what was not helpful, reflecting on personal coping processes and how these may affect expectations and responses in an intervention. Identification of any irresolution still present from prior losses needs to be made. Finally, by looking at one's own bereavement process, a psychotherapist can become aware of his or her personal limitations with respect to the kinds of clients and grief situations he or she is able to deal with. It is important to know the kinds of grieving persons that cannot be worked with, and when and how to make appropriate referrals when confronted with such clients.

DEATH AND BEREAVEMENT

Death is an inevitable part of the human experience. Through childhood, the awareness of death grows, bringing with it, in later childhood, fear and denial. During adolescence, death seems distant, almost impossible, when contrasted with growth and love. Thoughts of personal death tend to be set aside during the young adult years as the focus is on one's family and achievements. Yet death is ever-present and, during the middle years, it is glimpsed again, reminding the human being that time is not infinite. These reminders of death become more persistent and constant in the latter half of life. Death has its own time. As Raphael (1983) writes:

> It (death) may come when it is neither expected nor wanted. It is always unknown and unknowable, mystery and uncertainty. It may be peaceful or violent, anticipated or sudden, and it may be accompanied by stigma, shame, pain or pride. And it has the awesome power to rob one of those one loves — to bring the greatest of human pain, grief. (p. 4)

To work with those facing death and with the dying person's family members, it is critical that the psychotherapist have some knowledge of the dying and bereavement processes, and that he or she be encouraged to read in the field. The work of Elisabeth Kübler-Ross is well known and provides a place to begin.

Although there is criticism of Kübler-Ross's five stages in the journey of death, critics agree with her central theme: It is by drawing close to the dying and not fleeing from them that we discover what the dying person needs. That need may be for silence, for talk, for the freedom to weep or rage, for touch. Kübler-Ross (1969) urged a dialogue with the terminally ill, and her work, *On Death and Dying*, describes the relief provided to dying patients when invited to share their fears and needs on the journey toward death.

Kübler-Ross (1969) sees the process of dying as divided into five stages. Denial, she says, is the first response to the news of a fatal illness. "There must be some mistake! This cannot be!" Anger comes next, and the question is "Why me?" This anger may be expressed against doctors, family, God, fate or almost anything or anyone. Bargaining is the third response, an attempt to postpone the inevitable, promises made in exchange for more time. Depression, the fourth stage, is a sorrowing over past losses and a sorrowing for the great loss yet to come. Acceptance, the final stage, is not a time of "happiness" but rather one normally devoid of feelings, when the struggle is done, when there is no longer depression or fear or envy or anger, but rather a contemplation of the coming end "with a certain degree of quiet expectation."

While these stages are given as one way to understand the death journey, it must be understood that "stages" are more symbols of the experience that the dying individual may or may not go through than some lock-step process. The emotional states, the psychological mechanisms of defense, the needs and drives, are as variegated in the dying as they are in the non-dying. There are not five stages of dying; there are fifteen or fifty or 150.

In her beautiful book, *Endings and Beginnings* (1980), Sandra Albertson writes about the death of her husband, Mark:

> I asked Mark once if he had any sense of moving through the stages that Dr. Kübler-Ross described. He replied, "Yes, many times over." There is no lock-step progression from denial to acceptance. One is simply not angry at one point and then never angry again. You can not pull a patient kicking and screaming from stage one to stage five. (p. 124)

It is unfortunate that some have used the Kübler-Ross stages as if they were a rigid framework, a structure to be used to view the dying, and therefore have not seen the dying person as an individual. The stage theory gives little attention to an individual's particular illness, mode of treatment, environmental press, ethnicity and lifestyle. By focussing on the "stages," it is tempting to discount the dying person's very individual configuration of needs and resources.

The journey of emotional and social healing during bereavement is described by William Bridges in his book, *Transitions* (1980), and can be said to have three phases; the Ending phase which is the most traumatic and painful and in which the greater healing takes place; the Neutral Zone which is a time in between when one readjusts to the environment and establishes a new state of equilibrium, redefining the self; and New Beginnings when one moves back into the world forming new relationships.

This journey of healing takes between 18 months and 4 years to work through. Unfortunately, possibly because of implicit or explicit cultural attitudes, people tend to think that mourning should be over within a year and that the stages always follow in regular progression. People who have experienced bereavement will often say that this is not true and numerous studies confirm that the normal process of mourning and healing may be long and uneven. While the acute Ending phase usually lasts only several months, it may take several years for people to resume their normal level of activity and enjoy life again. And, in some ways, people are always changed by their experiences of loss. Albertson (1980) describes the process vividly:

> The journey out of grief is not a straight ascent, not some lock-step, linear process where sorrow can be crossed off like tasks completed. For a while, it may seem as if the same ground is being traveled over and over, the wound as raw and exposed, the loneliness and anguish as real as ever. Then the pattern becomes more like that of a spiral, where similar occasions, holidays, rememberings bring pain and sadness, but experienced at a less intense level. There are longer periods of quiet between. The days become not just a matter of coping, but filled with more and more pockets of gladness, self-confidence and hope. The initial panic of managing finances, children and home abates, as more alternatives and solutions become clear. The ache becomes less devastating, and one's mind is able to turn to topics other than death and one's own loss. The past family stops overwhelming the present, and one

can begin not only to hope for the future, but to be present in the moment, where one is. (p. 155)

As one goes through the bereavement journey, there are four tasks for mourning to be completed: (1) experiencing the pain of grief, (2) finding and utilizing a support system which will assist in the grieving and in adjustment to the environment after the loss, (3) handling practical matters which are present in any loss, and (4) accepting the reality of the loss and saying goodbye. This time of ending is often chaotic with great swings of emotions and no set pattern of movement. Behavior is erratic with emotional and physiological changes as well as changes in social relations. The experience differs greatly from person to person.

Typically, during the acute initial mourning, the bereaved report physical problems ranging from difficulty sleeping and eating to respiratory troubles and even pains and other symptoms that mimic those that the deceased person had experienced. The emotional experience, grief, is a normal but bewildering cluster of ordinary human emotions arising in response to the loss, commonly including sadness, anger, remorse, guilt, despair, anxiety, jealousy, aggression, and shame. Grief is an absolutely necessary and vital response to loss but is not predictable.

While most persons grieve in normal ways, there are those who, for a variety of reasons, do not, and thus their grieving could be characterized as abnormal. Four common abnormal grieving patterns are: (1) chronic grief reactions which are prolonged, excessive in duration and which never come to a satisfactory conclusion, (2) delayed grief reactions which are inhibited, suppressed or postponed, (3) exaggerated grief reactions which occur when the anxiety associated with the loss is exaggerated to the point of the development of a phobia or when the feelings of hopelessness become symptoms of irrational despair over a long period of time, and (4) masked or repressed grief reactions which often turn up as a physical symptom or maladaptive behavior such as delinquency.

Usually, emotional and physical complaints taper off and have no lasting consequences. However, some bereaved people are at increased risk for illness and even death. Bereavement can cause greater problems for those with existing illnesses and appears to have a role in precipitating new illness. Widowed men up to age 75 are about 1-1/2 times more likely to die than married men of the same age. Most bereaved people appear depressed for a few months; after one year, an estimated 10-20% of the widowed population is still sufficiently symptomatic to be considered clinically depressed.

As noted, support is a critical task in working through the ending of a loss. Social support has repeatedly been shown to be a reliable predictor of adjustment following a death. "People who have no support or feel they have no one to talk to are likely to do poorly" (Osterweis, 1985, p. 8). In order for the bereaved person to grieve effectively, support of family and friends is most important.

Bereavement generally occurs in the context of the family and affects the family system in many ways. Death of a family member means the family system is irrevocably changed. Death, therefore, is a crisis for the family unit as well as for each individual. The family's view of itself, the integrity of the family unit, the roles and responsibilities of family members, all change. After death, other family members will be in need of care. There may be competition for the roles of caregivers and for the role of "chief bereaved." Each member may feel the need for care and the need to grieve and mourn, but the system may only allow certain members such position and outlet.

Key to working through family issues regarding bereavement is openness of communication between members, thereby allowing for the sharing of information, expectations and grief. This openness is often difficult to achieve at the time of loss because each family member fears intensifying another's grief. Nevertheless, unless there is opportunity for mutual comfort and consolation, the mourning and healing processes may be blocked and resolution incomplete.

DYING AND OLD AGE

For the elderly, as has been stated earlier, bereavement is very much a part of life. While death may be experienced by a person of any age, for old people, losses occur much more frequently. For the institutionalized elderly in hospitals or long-term care facilities, death is all around. Robert Kastenbaum (1978) has noted that while

95% of those over 65 reside in noninstitutional settings, less than 1 in 5 die outside of an institution. Institutionalization is a part of our society's dying process. For the elderly, death of close friends, and even of many who are not particularly close, does not go unnoticed. Their deaths are at the very least constant reminders of the aging person's own mortality.

Every death has its own quality and importance just as does each relationship. The death of a spouse means multiple losses, not only the loss of a relationship, but loss of roles of the couple system, of a dream, and often loss of material security.

Today's elderly are often poorly equipped to deal with many of the daily tasks of living that must be taken on when a spouse dies. Older men and women were socialized to think in terms of a sharper division of labor than is the case with many younger persons. Elderly widows may know nothing of financial management; elderly widowers are likely to be equally unfamiliar with managing daily household routines. For both men and women, the loss of a spouse alters social relationships and precipitates feeling less comfortable and less welcome in couples-oriented activities. In addition, in marriages in which there has been high ambivalence, grieving seems to be complicated. Likewise, overly dependent relationships may result in bereavement reactions in which coping is particularly difficult.

The death of a sibling, regardless of emotional closeness or level of involvement in everyday activities, is a definite reminder of one's own mortality, and, if the sibling death has been the result of an inheritable disease, there is a heightened feeling of vulnerability. Sibling death often results in a change in the responsibilities among surviving children. For example, if the deceased was the one who took responsibility for keeping the family in contact with one another or had responsibility for caring for another family member, survivors will have to redistribute tasks. Because ambivalent feelings are common among siblings, the grieving process may be as complicated as it is for some spousal deaths.

Gower (1965) believes that "the most distressing and long-lasting of all griefs . . . is that for the loss of a grown child" (Osterwies, 1985, p. 11). With people living into their 80s and 90s, it is no longer unusual for some older people to outlive children as well as peers. The expectation is that of dying before one's children, and an adult child's death seems untimely and unfair. Bereaved elderly parents often exhibit heightened feelings of anger and guilt which have the potential for complicating the bereavement process. In addition to the emotional impact, an adult child's death may leave the elderly without a caretaker, thus necessitating major life-style changes.

Bereavement for the elderly is a potential source of major problems; the psychotherapist's awareness of bereavement issues will enable him to assist elderly persons more effectively.

THE PROCESS OF HELPING

As has been noted, the psychotherapist working with elderly clients must be open to the subjects of dying, death, and bereavement, and be able to deal with them, with awareness of the dying process and the issues of bereavement always tempered by knowledge of the individual's particular life configuration. For the elderly are as varied in their understanding and response to death as are those of any other age. At an older age, however, the reality of death is more sure and immediate. As Judith Viorst (1986) has written regarding the elderly and death, "Some speak of dying, some think of death, some suffer long enough to long for death, and others will deny and deny and deny, successfully persuading themselves that death will make an exception in their case" (p. 304).

In addition, a psychotherapist is wise to be on guard against equating "old" with "ready to die." It is a commonly held belief that old people are merely waiting for death. Robert Kastenbaum (1978) warns that if this attitude is present,

> . . . we can also hold our emotional responses and professional services within acceptable limits. . . . If we just *know* that death is appropriate for old people, then there is little need to explore precisely what this old man or woman is thinking or feeling. (p. 5)

Kastenbaum goes on to suggest that numerous commonly held attitudes about dying and death in old age are not supported by empirical evidence, but are nonetheless pervasive and can limit the ability of a psychotherapist to work with elderly clients. These attitudes include: the old person is "ready" if not actually "longing" to die; death is "natural" and "timely" for the old person; the "social loss" when an old person dies is minimal; memorialization and rituals associated with death are not of particular importance and may even extend the "morbid" aura of death over surrounding elders; and limited social and medical services should be applied to care of the young who still have life ahead of them.

These attitudes, along with the idea that the major developmental task of the elderly is to prepare for death, are hard to reconcile with increasing life expectancy of older persons and with the increasing importance given to the building of a productive and joyful old age and can unconsciously limit possibilities, even for the dying.

Unless the psychotherapist has been continually involved with the elderly person and the family through the dying process, it is unlikely that there will be involvement in the initial process of bereavement. However, in those cases where the therapist has been involved throughout the process, effective assistance can be provided to the bereaved. If there has been an on-going relationship, it is possible that the therapist would be involved in breaking bad news to the family. Usually the therapist, at this point, will be a part of the caregiving team and will provide support and continuing assistance. In breaking the news, the critical need is not simply to give information. It is important to find out what the family knows or imagines and to assess the capacity of the family to cope with the situation. Having taken an interest in the whole family throughout the dying process, the therapist will have built a trusting relationship which will make it easier to give the needed information. Having given that information, the therapist, as part of the caregiving team, needs to be prepared to stay with the family, giving them time and permission to react to the news.

There are three roles that a therapist can play in normal bereavement. The first is that of an interventionist. This initial role will occur in the earliest experience of bereavement, usually immediately after bad news has been given. It may continue for a few minutes or for several days. Intervention literally means "coming between" someone and their problems. In practical terms, that means stepping in, taking over, managing the bereaved person's affairs temporarily, and stepping out again when the need is past.

The goal of intervention is to assist the bereaved to take charge again as soon as possible, to regain mastery over their lives. Intervention often means assisting the bereaved to determine which decisions have priority and which ones can be delayed, which tasks must be undertaken by the primary bereaved and which can be done by others. Sensitivity to the family's own priorities and rules and not imposing the therapist's preferred patterns is of vital importance.

Comforting is also a part of this initial intervention. The appearance and behavior of a bereaved person is usually such as to evoke caring responses. The natural response is to hold, touch and to give sympathy. It may be that the therapist, at this point, may be hesitant, not able to touch, fearing it would break some personal barrier, create some inappropriate intimacy, or even constitute some form of assault. In these instances, it is best to offer comfort with a quiet and continuing presence, indicating preparation to stay with the bereaved until the initial shock has been absorbed and the bereaved can, in some way, reintegrate necessary defenses to cope with life tasks required. It is not unusual to find psychotherapists having difficulty offering this intervention and comfort since these responses represent a very personal human response, possibly going against a professional therapeutic style of detachment or disassociation that might be necessary at other times.

The second role for a therapist is that of support and consolation. The experience of a bereaved person, after the initial shock and numbness has passed, is to face and bear the pain of separation. The support/consolation role is to be with the bereaved person as needed, accepting the focus on the lost person and facilitating the bereaved's expression of yearning and protest, helping the bereaved to recognize the cause of distress; i.e., the absence of the dead person. This means being a listening presence, comfortable with silence; bearing pain and confusion with the bereaved; responding with encouragement to the expression of strong feelings such as anger; and lending strength when there is need for an emotional "prop." It requires willingness to suspend the impulse toward premature comfort as a way of helping the bereaved ward off pain. It means "listening without judging, hearing without retreating, evoking without forcing, and understanding without condescend-ing" (Mitchell & Anderson, 1983, p. 117).

This supportive relationship begins at the time of the death and will continue for several weeks through the initial experience of grieving. It is important to realize that support offered at this time does not stop the bereaved's feelings of loss. Rather, it can help the bereaved know, name, and express the pain caused by the absence of the person who has died.

The third therapy role is that of facilitating acceptance of the finality of the loss. Emotional release from attachment to the dead person is essential for healing. One gains emotional release from the lost person by actively incorporating the experiences of the rela-tionship into memory. Reminiscing or remembering with another person is the principal means by which such a memory is built and strengthened. Shared memories help the bereaved gain needed emo-tional distance from the past. Usually this therapy role is carried out several weeks after the death when the initial grief reaction has tempered, although the process of remembering may begin natu-rally shortly after a death such as at the time of the funeral. The therapist's role is to facilitate the acceptance of finality through the review of both negative and positive aspects of the lost relationship, and the expression of affects that this evokes. The therapist can both facilitate this acceptance process and directly encourage the be-reaved person's support group to do so.

Remembering can be a painful process that is not easily begun. The therapist may need to give gentle but insistent encouragement toward remembering, an insistence that may be experienced as con-frontation. To insist that the bereaved actively create memories rather than shutting them away particularizes the memory of what was lost. This remembering is painful because it brings to aware-ness the complicated mixture of emotions connected with the lost person, but there is no other way through mourning.

These three roles for the therapist in normal bereavement are im-portant whether the bereaved is a spouse or a child of the person who died. During this time, it is important that the therapist "name" behaviors and the loss experience clearly. To say "die," "dead," and "death" is to name the loss and it models an important behavior to the bereaved who may want to run from the reality of the loss.

Most bereavement is normal and, as indicated, the helping role is less therapeutic than it is supportive. Therapeutic assistance is most beneficial among bereaved persons who perceive their families as unsupportive or who, for other reasons, are thought to be at special risk (Worden, 1982, p. 52).

It is important for the therapist, therefore, to be able to assess the situation of the bereaved in order to evaluate the level of risk and provide the most effective help. Raphael (1983) has developed a therapeutic assessment designed to explore a number of areas of grief. She believes that the framework provided by the assessment provides a "risk profile" for bereaved persons and delineates specific areas where there may be difficulties. Specific crisis or short-term bereavement counseling may then be provided in the first weeks or months following the loss. Where there is indication that bereavement is taking a pathological course, more extensive psychotherapy will be indicated.

The questions used by Raphael (1983) in this therapeutic assessment are:

1. Can you tell me a little about the death? What happened? What happened that day? (Raphael believes that the bereaved's capacity to talk about the death and the pattern of emotional responsiveness about it will start to become obvious as the bereaved discusses this question.)
2. Can you tell me about him(her), about your relationship from the beginning? (This question enhances the remembering and provides a therapist with a history of the relationship. It may reveal the quality of the relationship and the level of ambivalence and dependence involved. The therapist will be able to more clearly assess the degree to which the bereaved is denying the loss, provide information on the progress of mourning and relinquishment of the lost relationship, and may be able to assess the grief affects associated with mourning such as levels of sadness, anger, particular guilts or abnormal levels of guilt.)
3. What has been happening since the death? How have things

been with you and your family and friends? (Raphael uses this question to assess evidence of risk factors such as perceived inadequacy of social support or other crises or stresses that may have occurred. Indication of blocks to resolution or a delayed, inherited or distorted pattern of bereavement may be assessed.)

4. Have you been through any other bad times like this recently or when you were young? (This question, according to Raphael, enables evaluation of earlier losses and seeks specifically for signs of any other concurrent crises or stressors and their effects as possible risk factors for bereavement resolution.) (pp. 362-367)

Any bereavement therapy has, as its primary goal, the encouragement of grieving and facilitation of the mourning process to promote emotional and social health. Particular goals may be developed for each individual and should reflect the bereaved person's risk profile. The therapeutic relationship at this time usually develops quickly as the bereaved is highly motivated to seek help for relief of the distress. This therapeutic experience should be short-term and focussed on the previously-mentioned goals.

Where there is an abnormal pattern of bereavement, longer-term therapy may be indicated. A variety of therapeutic models may be used. Raphael (1983) defines a process of Focal Psychotherapy, "involving an assessment of the particular form of pathological bereavement response and management specific to it as well as to the etiological processes involved," with its goal being "the conversion of the response to a more normal pattern in which the patient is able to grieve and mourn" (p. 375). Worden (1982) has found Gestalt therapy, especially use of the "empty chair" technique as helpful, with the patient talking directly to the deceased person in the present tense (p. 74). Re-grief therapy, as developed initially by Volkan, is another model with two specific outcomes sought, helping the patient to understand why mourning has not been able to be completed, thus assisting in that completion, and helping the bereaved to experience and express the grieving emotions (Raphael, 1983, pp. 385-386).

Other models, including a variety of behavioral therapy approaches, can be used in working with the bereaved. With any technique, timing is essential. It is crucial that the therapist know how to time interventions. The encouragement of affect before a patient is ready is not appropriate, and ill-timed interventions will not work.

It is important that, in addition to dealing with the bereaved individual, family aspects of bereavement be dealt with. Family systems may assist in the process of bereavement, or they may actively interfere with grief. Family members will grieve at different times and in different ways which may lead to friction, further pain, and misunderstanding. It is important to remember that, after the loss, the family system as a whole is hurt and wounded.

There are several goals in working with families at the time of bereavement. Because family members often find it difficult, at first, to show their feelings and concerns to one another following death, family work would help with simple, open, and honest communication about the "facts of the death," again, "naming" the loss and not avoiding discussion. The work should also emphasize the sharing of feelings of family members which may involve different experiences of each person in the weeks and months that follow the death. The work may also involve facilitating review of the lost relationship in its positive and negative aspects.

The well-trained psychotherapist who is knowledgeable about dying, death and bereavement can support the elderly person's experience of aging and death and can facilitate the healing processes of bereavement in family members.

REFERENCES

Albertson, S. H. (1980). *Endings and beginnings*. New York: Ballantine Books.

Bridges, W. (1980). *Transitions: Making sense of life's changes*. Reading, MA: Addison-Wesley.

Buskingham, R. W. (1983). *The complete hospice guide*. New York: Harper and Row.

Dunlop, R. S. (1978). *Helping the bereaved*. Bowie, MD: The Charles Press.

Kastenbaum, R. (1978). Death, dying and bereavement in old age: New developments and their possible implications for psychosocial care. *Aged Care & Services Review, 1*(3), pp. 1-10.

Kübler-Ross, E. (1969). *On Death and Dying*. New York: Macmillan.

Mitchell, K. R., & Anderson, H. (1983). *All our losses, all our griefs: Resources for pastoral care*. Philadelphia: The Westminster Press.

Osterweis, M. (1985). Bereavement and the Elderly. *Aging*, 348.

Parkes, C. M., & Weiss, R. S. (1983). *Recovery from bereavement*. New York: Basic Books.

Raphael, B. (1983). *The anatomy of bereavement*. New York: Basic Books.

Viorst, J. (1986). *Necessary losses*. New York: Simon & Schuster.

Worden, W. J. (1982). *Grief counseling and grief therapy: A handbook for the mental health practitioner*. New York: Springer Publishing.

Weizman, S. G., & Kamm, P. (1987). *About mourning: Support and guidance for the bereaved*. New York: Human Services Press.

Aging and Family Therapy:
A Final Note

George A. Hughston
Victor A. Christopherson
Marilyn J. Bonjean

Psychotherapy for the elderly and their families requires the services of different types of practitioners working together as a problem-oriented team. It is our hope that the papers contained in this collection will assist with the awareness of a variety of issues implicit to family caregiving and assistance to the elderly.

The papers in this collection have focussed on problem areas related to old age and the effects age-related changes have upon families. All papers responded to the systemic nature of the family as members interact with one another and with society. By design, materials have been presented which emphasize potentially difficult areas and offer solutions and resources which should contribute to the development of additional systemic intervention strategies of benefit to clients.

Just ten years ago, systemic intervention was not widely practiced by family therapists, and only recently has it become important and well recognized by those working specifically with the elderly. This collection combines gerontology and family therapy for the first time.

Major demographic trends in the United States present ever-increasing numbers and percentages of old people, with those 75 years-of-age and older, the "old-old," increasing in numbers most rapidly. This group constitutes a focal problem for many families, and these are the issues to which many of the papers in this collection respond. Multi-generational family strategies are required in order to prepare for the uncertain futures of individuals in this age group. As a "count down" begins, there is no substitute for knowledge of alternatives by those involved in caregiving services. A great deal of insight and interpersonal competence, particularly from adult children, is required for a family to maximize its abilities to function as an effective system. Conflict from many sources is inevitable; past unresolved interpersonal issues, demands of caregiving time and money, misinterpretations or reactions to sensory loss, modifications in status, and perhaps changes in cognition and perception may interact to create family chaos. The services of a skilled family psychotherapist will become increasingly important for prolongation of effective functioning among the aged and their families.

Although the multiple issues implicit in family caregiving of the aged are complex, they must sooner or later by addressed by policy at the national level. Rewards must encourage family assistance of the aged. Tax breaks, for example, could encourage family involvement. Until that day, however, it will be increasingly incumbent upon therapists and other professional practitioners to increase the armamentarium of their skills to enable them to more effectively deal with the problems within the family system. These papers were designed with this purpose in mind.